How to Flirt With Women

A Seduction Guide to Attract Beautiful Girls
with your Personality.

How to Sustain a Captivating Conversation and
Create a Deep Connection with Her.

(Step-by-Step Exercises)

Table of Content

Introduction

Did you know that around 90 percent of all communication occurs non-verbally and the fairer sex is extremely good at picking and reading body language signals you're giving? Yes, seems like a scary prospect. However, use it right, and you can brilliantly turn this into an alpha male super-power. These are tons of other secret tips are yours for the taking with this handy resource of a book that spills the beans on being the ultimate girl magnet, who has them eating out of your hands.

Did you know that experts have stated that even when you are dating, the verbal language is often relegated to subordinate status? It's the non-verbal communication or body language that gains prominence. We have covered tons of strategies on impressing women with killer body language. Women are instinctive creatures, who demonstrate far greater awareness than men think. They are super efficient when it comes to deciphering both verbal and non-verbal cues, even if you are stating just the opposite of it. Scary again? You bet! That's why it is said that it is tough to fool a woman and probably even tougher to know what she wants.

This means if you are saying you are totally into someone, but your body language reveals otherwise, women are not likely to believe what you say.

Ever realized why sometimes even the most average looking men are natural chick magnets, who have women flocking to them like moths.

There's got to be something that they are doing right. They are just ordinary guys with extraordinary charisma and communication skills.

Their personality creates a hypnotic, magnetic charm that attracts women by the dozen.

What are these powerful secrets that are the key to winning a woman's heart and getting her in bed? Is it only confidence, independence, charisma or another collection of "x" factors or mojo?

I'll let you in on a little secret that can be used to your advantage. Most men possess a body language that screams "I am absolutely used to the idea of being liked and received by the opposite sex. Run miles away from me."

The reality is that owning an appealing personality will make you stand out from the average Joes struggling with confidence, communication, and persona. Truth be told –a majority of men give out terrible, desperate and unattractive clues, something that drives women miles away from them. Terrible as it sounds, they come across as plain desperate. There, you've spotted a loophole already and can gain an edge by learning the finer nuances of impressing your dream woman with a seductive personality.

Do you know the number one reason why men fail to build a dating and sex life of their dreams? They just don't have a clue about how to take action and charm women they desire. They are unable to overpower their compelling fear of rejection. They are weighing themselves under the weight of how to be good enough for the woman. Men want to kiss, seduce, capitulate with women, without having a clue about how to be a man a woman just can't resist.

In reality, seduction is an art and science. They are several subtle body languages and scientific mind tricks that can be used to make yourself absolutely irresistible to women. From persuasion through gestures and expressions to actions that make you come across as completely irresistible, this book has plenty of little-known strategies and secret tips that will put you on the highway to being the ultimate alpha male. There are plenty of psychological techniques that can be used to attract desirable women if you know how to play them in the right way.

Alpha males use unbelievably stealthy seduction tricks that help them make really bold and fast moves. One minute you'll spot him talking to a woman, the next moment they will get into a cab heading to her home. The man's actions are appealing simply because he is aware of how to behave around attractive women. These men know exactly how to display the perfect body language, listen to women, how to touch women in the right way, and build just the right measure of sexual tension.

To enhance your individual personality, you must work towards making it what you want, and then imbibe it as an almost subconscious part of your everyday existence. It will be one of the things that come most naturally to you when you present yourself in front of women.

Personality, charm, confidence and body language plays on a very scientific and subconscious level. When you are positive and confident, the subconscious mind receives signals of being confident, self-assured and in control.

The brain quickly recognizes these body language clues as a sign of unwavering confidence, and later directs the body (gestures, posture, expressions, movement) to behave in a more confident and self-assured manner. Thus it's a cycle, the subconscious mind is led to believe that you are confident person, which it reinforces through non-verbal signals that reveal even more confident, in control behavior. And nothing is more irresistible for a woman than a man who is comfortable and confident in his skin.

Use the examples, secret strategies and subtle seduction techniques discussed in the book to send the right non-verbal signals to women. Of course, you won't go from being a struggling Joe to the ultimate alpha male in a day. However, with time, impressing women will become a second skin.

Fasten your seatbelts, and get ready for an enjoyable adventure that trains you to pick-up the ultimate techniques and strategies to woo your dream woman.

Chapter One:

Brilliant Strategies for Building an Unforgettable First Impression

Let's face a bitter, hard truth about life. Some guys have it naturally easier than others when it comes to attracting women. They just have it in them.

These are the dudes who always bag the champion's trophy, while lesser mortals are left struggling with consolation prizes like boys' night outs and Netflix binge-watching sessions.

It can drive you crazy. You want to know "what are these dudes doing that I am not doing?" Of course, it's understandable for that Greek god incarnates, rich, sophisticated family background, flashy cars, and perfect jobs. However, what about the several average Joes who seem to score really well when it comes to wooing woman (almost as if they have access to some secret, magic potion).

I actually know several seeming boring, average guys, who don't even possess unusual talents (other than attracting women which is the best if you ask me) draw women like magnets. What's it about them that they make such a positive impression on women and keep bagging dates with them over and over again until they get hitched. I mean wow!

I dug really deep into the subject and realized that it isn't just a single subject but a combination of areas of study including psychology, evolutionary sciences, neurology, attraction/sexuality and much more. You could write a thousand books about what a woman wants and it'd still be less, which is why I am sharing the best and most effective tips I've learned and mastered over the years, minus the mediocrity and fluff.

Here are some magnificent tips for being the ultimate first impression rock star.

1. Maintain an Easy and Relaxed Posture

A woman doesn't want to see her potential mate going all jittery and sweaty at the prospect of striking a conversation with her. Stay relaxed, calm, lean against a bar wall, hold your glass on the side (and not front) and other similar postures/gestures that convey a more relaxed, unruffled and confident demeanor.

Women don't like to see men get all worked up about something as harmless (well at least they perceive it that way) as talking to a woman. In their mind, if he gets rattled by such innocuous things, how he is going to help her through the storm?

If you are relaxed and confident, the woman is likelier to feel more relaxed and at ease in your company too.

2. Avoid Playing Interviewer

Instead of going all FBI on her and inquiring where she lives, what are her leisure pursuits, and what her neighbor's dog ate for dinner last night, make a classy yet definitive comment about her. For instance, "you have the quintessential Chicago vibe" or "you must be a financial consultant."

This is a great strategy for preventing the conversation from slipping into a rut. Also, even if you are wrong in making the definitive statements, she'll admire your confidence. So it's actually a win-win. If you say the right thing, you've wowed her with your perceptiveness. If your guess is wrong, she'll be wowed by the attitude.

Try this technique next time you're trying to impress women at a bar.

3. Place a Mental Speed Breaker

As soon as a woman agrees to have you seated next to her or starts talking to you, don't assume she's game or suggestive, flirty or innuendo-filled talks. She may very well be seeking an engaging and meaningful conversation.

Don't try to push things hard so she'll back off. You'll do nothing but trigger her protective gear and shut her off from any further conversation.

Guys make the mistake of moving too fast after a woman offers them a genuine compliment or a full-throated laugh to their jokes.

She may be shy, reserved, and may not too kindly to you forcing things upon her.

Even if she doesn't laugh or respond positively on the face of it, don't automatically assume that he doesn't like you. Some people just take more time, meetings and space to know others.

Don't overstep into her comfort zone in order to impress her. Just give her the time to figure you out and you'll do well.

4. Let Your Real Personality Shine

Women are naturally attracted to men who aren't afraid of revealing their real selves, irrespective of what others may think about them. There's something irresistible about people who have the courage to put their true selves in front of others regardless of other's opinions.

The lure of someone who embraces who they really are is hard for women to overlook. For instance, you're trying hard to impress a woman and she says she isn't into baseball at all. You then downplay your own interest in baseball in order to prevent upsetting her or winning her favor. Women are quick to notice when you aren't being true to yourself or you suddenly change your stance and downplay things you were upbeat about a minute ago.

This doesn't help you earn brownie points with your crush. Come across as someone who isn't afraid of being their true self in front of people. When you are true to yourself, it automatically conveys to the woman that you absolutely have it in you to be true to others too.

It reveals less deceit, and a more open, genuine and straightforward personality. Being true to yourself is at the base of integrity, which is what almost every woman is seeking in her man.

Don't worry about the woman not seeing you as a likely match. You aren't Siamese twins joined at the hip. There can be different interests, likes, and hobbies. The positives far outweigh the negatives.

When you both are your real self, it's so much easier to be with each other in the long run, isn't it? You don't have to try to convince someone about being something you aren't. It's too much pressure and can be tricky in the long run.

The dynamics of two unique and individual personalities coming together is much more interesting than trying to ape each other.

A relationship where both have the freedom to pursue their individual interests, while also sharing a few common goals is always healthy over one where the partner is desperately trying to be something to fit the other's expectations.

Just as men appreciate a woman who is her own person, a woman doesn't fancy men who hang on to every word they utter. They like men who have a mind of their own, rather than those who are dying to be accepted.

5. Be Confident Without Being Pompous

Women can sniff the difference between confidence and brag from miles away. Their sense of decoding the intention behind every action is marvelously high. Their strong intuitive powers make it easy for women to know the intent behind an act.

Clichéd as it may sound, women dig confident and self-assured men. It's all about mind over matter. When two equally talented players are playing against each other, the one looks confident and plays more aggressively has a definite advantage, at least in the eyes of the onlooker.

Before a woman judges you on other factors, she is subconsciously assessing your confidence levels. And confidence is not equal bragging to her. Even though women dig wealthy, well-settled men with great jobs, they are seldom attracted to dudes who brag about it.

Bragging in their mind triggers a sort of red alert that the guy is low on confidence. A truly confident, self-assured and self-respecting man doesn't need to spell out his achievements or assets. Women understand that the need to boast originates from a faulty self-confidence mechanism.

Next time when you meet an interesting woman you want to create a favorable first impression on, narrate an interesting story that lets her figure out on her own that you're successful and popular.

6. Be an Expert at Catching Trigger Words

Now, this isn't very easy to explain but a massively powerful strategy nevertheless to get a woman to notice you. Take any regular conversation that you can have with a woman.

For instance, if the woman mentions that she's attending a friend's bachelorette party pick a trigger word and cash in on it. Use the most commonly heard stereotype about the trigger word (bachelorette party in this case). So let's say hunky male strippers.

As soon as she mentions, she's attending her friend's bachelorette party, grab the clue and instead of a bland response like "that's amazing" say something like, "Amazing!

I was looking out for your girl squad. I am the exotic and hot male stripper you ordered tonight." Makes the conversation so much zingier and memorable.

Have lots of other interesting things handy to talk about. An exciting conversationalist is hard to forget. Narrate stories of interesting people you've met. Share interesting bits about yourself that she may not know yet. By revealing a bit of vulnerability a man makes himself highly irresistible to a woman.

7. Offer a Sincere Compliment

Compliments are wonderful ice breakers if done right. If pay her a sincere and well-thought compliment, she will find it tough to ignore you. Think about her best features or qualities. Of course, don't focus too much on her physical aspects (she may have a low figure but now is not the time to mention it).

Keep the compliment short, detailed and genuine. It can really backfire if it borders on plain flattery to win favors. Instead, focus on something that people rarely notice such as I love the way you've worn that shirt or I really like the way you gesticulate while talking or you've got a very commanding voice. This shows her you are paying attention beyond the obvious and that you're keenly noticing things being missed by others. Don't wax opera style eloquence while paying a compliment? Keep it short to retain its impact.

Wording the compliment carefully is as important as delivering it a right compliment. Instead of saying something like, "that's a fabulous outfit you're wearing" say something like "you look really nice in that outfit." Focus on the woman, not on the outfit. Smile your sincerest best while saying it, make eye contact (which reveals you really mean it and not simply putting them on) and keep your body language confident.

8. Treat People Respectfully and Compassionately

Yes, a woman's antenna is unfortunately always up when she's seizing up potential mates just about anywhere. If you want to really score with her, treat everyone around respectfully and kindly.

A bad, arrogant and brash attitude just won't cut with most women. How a man treats people who can do little for him in return is very indicative of his general nature and personality.

Do not walk around like you own the place and treat others contemptuously. Never patronize or talk down to people in her presence (or even otherwise duh!). Women don't view you in parts. They can't digest the fact that you're uber chivalrous with them while treating someone else with absolute disdain.

They are sharp at perceiving intentions and notice just about all your actions with a secret magnifying glass (scary I know).

The best way to deal with this is to be nice, polite, respectful and kind towards everyone.

They will quickly gather they can expect similar behavior from you in a future relationship.

9. Prepare a Few Killer Opening Lines

There are volumes and volumes dedicated to the perfect opening like or pick-up line.

Frankly, it puts too much pressure on guys to deliver the perfect opening pitch.

The best way to handle it is to avoid stressing over it. Please avoid cheesy pick-up lines like, "I bet you are a vegetable because you're a cute-cumber" or "Do you have a pen? I just want to write our beautiful future?" or "Are you sure you aren't appendix because I really want to take you out?" Trust me, you won't see them again.

Just pick something that sounds cheeky, open-ended and lively. Be creative you're your lines, they should be uniquely you.

Borrowing hackneyed and stolen lines makes you come across as a person who lacks imagination, which is certainly not something women want in their prospective partners.

Deliver it with unshakable confidence, even if you have absolutely no idea about what you're saying. Confidence alone will help you steer the conversation in the direction you want it to.

However, holding command over a conversation without the other person realizing that you are controlling it is an art that needs to be practiced.

Don't give her the impression that you are leading the conversation.

Use the trick car salesmen are trained to use to impress their customers.

They are trained to look for clues about what the customer is carrying in his car and strike a conversation based on it.

For instance, if they spot a golf kit in the customer's car, that's a clue for the salesman to strike up a conversation about golf. So he may say something like, "I am just learning to play golf" or "did you watch last night's game? Similarly, if someone has a full camping kit, they may drop a line about camping over the weekend.

Replicate the car salesman tactic with the woman you're trying to impress. Look around or clues about what she is wearing, carrying, etc. When you spot something significant, dive head-on into the topic and start chatting casually about it.

Women aren't impressed when they get the feeling that you're trying to impress them. Keep it more casual and chatty to win their trust, and get to know them better.

10. Get Rid of the Dancing Monkey Syndrome

Several guys fall prey to the dancing monkey syndrome while trying to make a favorable first impression on a woman. The dancing money syndrome is nothing but trying too hard to be funny or entertaining. Hold yourself back, and be a bit of challenge for the woman. Don't jump around all over the place trying to make her laugh.

A woman shouldn't really get the impression that you're trying to snag every available hot chick's number at the bar or anywhere else. If you present yourself more frivolously, they'll take you less seriously. Once she gathers the attention of every woman present there, she's less likely to respond to your overtures. Demonstrate that you are only seeking the right ladies.

Chapter Two:

Body Language Tips to Sweep Women Off Their Feet

Did you know people meeting you for the first time form an impression about you in the initial four seconds? Hard truth? You bet! If you want to go from being a weekend Netflix binge-watcher to a guy who is never short of dates, you got to be a dude who creates a stellar first impression. If there's one secret sauce or magic potion when it comes wooing a woman, it is creating a powerful initial impression.

Deep research into the science of seduction reveals that it attracts isn't confined to a single domain. It is a combination of neurology (NLP), psychology, sexual studies, and evolutionary science, which is why I am revealing the ten most super awesome tips when it comes to sweeping a woman off her feet in the first meeting.

1. Grab Your Place under the Spotlight

Guess what, even though we have evolved from our primitive existence, our subconscious mind is still deeply hard-wired in its patterns when it comes to relationships and social gestures. There's a reason we still mark our territory physically and subconsciously, and entering our space leads us to act in a more territorial manner.

Well okay, no one's asking you to grab the limelight by acting weird or hyper-energetic. One way to demonstrate confidence when meeting a woman you desire for the first time is to take your own space. Don't be the nerd who fades into the background, while others hog center stage.

You don't want to stand out for the wrong reason but that doesn't mean you don't get noticed (which is equally bad if you ask me).

Own your zone and take up your space immediately. Expert tip for owning your space – seize up space within 3 feet as your own private space. Think of yourself as owning that private bubble and ensuring any woman who passes through it has a great time. Focus on completely owning the space around you, and you'll have the gathering's hottest gals noticing you.

Somebody language and seduction experts suggest taking as much space as you can. If you are seated in the lobby, lean behind and spread out your legs. This is a subconscious, territorial instinct that women notice. Well, in the woman's mind, if you are occupying a lot of "territory", you are the room's alpha male. The one who is in command, as well as fun, confident and laid-back.

2. Create an Emotional Rapport

The journey from meeting a woman to taking her to bed becomes surprisingly easy when you build a powerful emotional rapport with her. Psychologically, mirroring is one of the most effective ways to forge a strong mental connection with the woman you desire. Start mirroring the way she stands, speaks, holds her glass and gesticulates.

Keep it discreet and don't make it look like you are raping her. Subconsciously, mirroring sends the other person a message that you are pretty much like them and makes it easier for them to connect with you on a mental plane. Gradually mimic her posture or use the same words/phrases as she does. Once you practice this strategy, it will come effortlessly.

For example, if the woman holds her glass on her left side, try and hold your glass of drink on the left side too. If they are making a particular gesture with their hands, try and make that gesture too for conveying that you identify with what they are trying to communicate, and acknowledging the same.

Mirroring works wonderfully well because it is seen as something that's beyond the realm of our conscious awareness. When you repeat someone's actions and words, you are secretly sending signals of familiarity to them through the subconscious.

Seduction boy language experts suggest that you should mirror or mimic a specific gesture three seconds after it is first noticed. This lets you imitate a person without them freaking out or becoming suspicious about your behavior. Although on the face of it, you are simply mirroring the lady's body language, the end goal is to match her feelings, views, thoughts and yes – maybe even the breathing pattern. Even minor actions like posture, expressions, blinking, verbal acknowledgments, and scratching should be matched. If this technique is implemented correctly, the woman will be falling like you like a pack of cards!

Another quick way to build an emotional rapport is to reveal a vulnerability in the correct manner. According to research, some women are taken in by weaker men. However, weakness is also a relative trait. Remember to never make the blunder of revealing low value and terrible weaknesses. This may really go against you. For example, you may want to narrate a sob story related to your ex, but this will only make you look like a cry baby who cannot move on.

If you are using this psychological trick, ensure you pick your weaknesses with care and don't opt for weaknesses that make you look low-value or unflattering. Instead of concentrating on your past, build emotional rapport via future projections. How about an exciting thing you've fantasizing about all along? Talk about an exciting travel experience that's on the top of your bucket list. Just reveal some fun thing without overdoing it. You are doing nothing but controlling the woman's mind without making her realize.

Women possess way more powerful and vivid imagination than men, which makes them see the exciting things in their mind's eye. Also, you've shared a personal dream or goal with her, which makes you instantly adorable to her. Practice this technique regularly, and keep watching for the body language of couples who are already in the rapport building stage. You'll witness amazing results in little time.

3. Open Up

You don't want the woman of your dreams to think you're a closed, secretive and guarded person. Of course, you don't want to come across as a sparrow on steroids, but keeping an open and approachable demeanor works to create a glowing first impression.

I'll let you in on all secret body language strategies to appear warm, open and approachable. To begin with, keep your palms facing upwards (open and exposed). Remember, how you reveal all your cards by flashing your palms upwards in a game? Well, you aren't exactly revealing all your cards here. However, you are demonstrating a more "open to you baby" kind of demeanor.

Another big cross on the list of things to avoid is crossing your legs or arms while standing or sitting. Even if you don't realize, it has "closed" written on it in bold. You are psychologically blocking yourself from your wonder woman.

Another vehement no-no, if you're holding a drink, don't hold it right in front of you. Hold the glass down, sideways.

Master these little known techniques that most men don't have a clue about to enjoy an edge over them when it comes to garnering attention from the opposite sex.

Hide your feelings by all means but, but keep the hands open. Also, displaying a lightly off the limits or playing hard to get body language doesn't hurt. You need to keep a fine balance between not acting too distant (will make it appear you aren't interested) and not acting too eager (which makes you come across as desperate).

According to research conducted by Timothy Wilson and Erin Whitchurch of the University of Virginia, acting slightly indifferent towards women can lead them to contemplate your distant behavior, and eventually, develop a liking for you.

4. Be Attentive

Women don't take it kindly if they are relegated to secondary status. If you fancy them, they should be the center of your attention. Don't move around or act fidgety around a woman you desire. Preoccupation and distraction is a huge turn-off. You're not giving off a very flattering vibe to the object of your desire if you make perpetually fidgeting and nervous gestures. A man who is in control of his body language will be taken more seriously than one who is awkward with his gestures and movements. Keep your feet slightly apart while sitting, which will prevent you from constantly shifting your weight from one side to another.

Shifty, fidgety and distracted gestures are a huge sign of nervousness that takes away from an essentially calm, confident and relaxed demeanor, which you want to portray.

Don't make too many confusing gestures that send the woman you desire perplexing non-verbal signals. Twitching your body excessively or making too many animated hand gestures is an absolute no-no. It gives off the feeling that you aren't very comfortable with your body and leaves a damp first impression. When you appear uncomfortable with your own body, how do you expect women to be comfortable near you?

Of course, you don't have to be all over the woman and shower her with unwanted attention. That's a huge no-no too. Acting a little indifferent to things happening around you is alright; just don't act too fidgety and distracted. Cool indifference is mighty appealing, nervousness is not.

A majority of men falter here. They believe it's cool to act all busy and distracted to impress a woman. So, what does Mr. X do? Whip out a smartphone from his pocket and pretend to occupy with important matters. What does it reveal to the lady? You're simply not interested enough to give her undivided attention. Well, don't blame her for getting the impression that you want to be somewhere else.

Instead of appearing distracted, keep all objects of distraction away and appear interested in your immediate surroundings. Keep your body language alert, focused and aware of your environment. Put your head up, and relish the moment, which makes you appear more approachable. Plus, you pick up all the silent, non-verbal invitations/signals women stealthily send you.

If you really want to score with a woman, avoid showing too much emotion or reaction to things happening around you in the first meeting. Display a more unaffected demeanor. Let others play the guessing game about how you think and feel. This makes the challenge of getting to know you up, close and personal even more compelling.

Stay at the top of your dating/seduction game by showing you are always in control and relaxed. Everyone loves people who own the situation.

5. Flaunt the Sexiest Voice You Can

Ever wondered why woman are attracted like moths to a fireball by men with deep, husky and low-pitched voices? Women are essentially auditory creatures who are instantly attracted to a calm, strong and controlled voice/tone.

Talk too fast and you'll come across as nervous. Speak slowly, and you'll run the risk of appearing dumb. Keep your tone steady, unwavering and well-paced. Make a conscious effort to make yourself audience and clear by speaking slower than you usually do while talking to a woman. It will award you greater control of what you're saying (plus you'll time to think about what you're going to say next).

Avoid stressing about mistakes and stammering during the conversation. Even if you do make a mistake while speaking, cover it up by saying something humorous quickly to salvage the situation. Think and speak according to the situation.

Something like, "Ah! Damn, this is exactly what happens when you're in the company of sweepingly attractive women. You totally forget what you want to say." This will not just be flattering to the lady but also make you come across as high on wit and humor. Self-deprecating humor is a sign of huge confidence.

Sometimes while talking, pause for a moment and appear serious. This creates an aura of power, influence, and confidence.

6. Keep a Relaxed Posture

Get this straight and clear, women absolutely don't dig men who go all nervous and jittery at the idea of introducing themselves to women. Nervousness is the biggest first impression killer.

Stay calm, relaxed and in control to create a magnificent first impression. Ensure the smallest gestures (often subconscious) such as holding your glass (hold it sideways and not in front) and standing (leaning against a wall is incredibly sexy) appear relaxed.

Leaning back will up your game like no other. When you are in a sitting or standing pose, simply lean back and look relaxed. This open and inviting gesture demonstrates that you're warm and approachable. Added tip – Let your arms loose by the side. Avoid leaning forward and crossing your arms.

It shows a more closed, protected and shielded approach, where you are not open to being approached by strangers. Play smooth by sitting back in a relaxed posture, and you'll appear totally in control and approachable.

It indicates to the woman that you aren't trying too hard to impress, and are an extremely confident and self-assured individual. To women, it isn't a huge deal to approach them and talk to them. If you get rattled about something as non-fuss (in their eyes) as this, it indicates that you are incapable of handling bigger challenges.

I'll let you in on a cool secret. I know most men are a bundle of nerves in front of women they fancy. To keep yourself calm, relaxed (and almost Zen-like), practice taking slow, relaxed breaths focused on the belly. Witness your stomach rising and falling as you take well-defined, slow and deep breaths. Don't take tensed, rushed breaths into the lungs. This tightens your muscles and makes your overall body language appear tensed and nervous.

Give your muscles an opportunity to relax. Once the stress and tension alleviate, it is easier to radiate natural confidence. Your body will be shinning with a fresh lease of confidence, and women will invariably be attracted to you.

Do not slump over or slouch while approaching a woman or introducing yourself to someone for the first time. She'll be shooting in another direction before you finish saying hello. Slumping, crossing arms and looking at the floor will kill your chances of creating a positive first impression. It isn't a very appealing stance, especially when you're meeting someone for the first time, and reflects low confidence and a more negative attitude.

Always hold yourself high physically and mentally. Pull back your shoulders, and keep your head straight up. Act like you're a man who deserves a woman's affection, admiration, and attention. Women (or for that matter) find people who know their true worth absolutely irresistible.

Women feel more at ease in the company of men who are relaxed, self-assured and confident about themselves.

7. Walk the Talk

Well, what's that we've heard about don't walk like you own the world, walk like you don't care who does! Walk with your head held down, and you've ruined it even before beginning.

When you walk in with your hands tucked inside the pocket, man do you look completely off limits or unapproachable. Leave your hands dangling sideways, keep your back erect and tilt your head slightly. Next, stick out your chest, and draw your shoulders firmly back. This again reveals natural confidence.

Have you ever observed a millionaire or a celebrity? They are almost always walking exactly as described above, radiating confidence that's hard to ignore.

There's a powerful and commanding aura each time they enter a room. That is the kind of arresting attention you want to attract from women.

A man's walking style since primitive times is subconsciously viewed as him approaching a woman for the purpose of mating. Taking firm, confident and well-paced strides is a sign of someone who knows what he wants and how to get it.

Take, for instance, you're in a store and fancy a girl. What is the best way to approach her? Walk confidently towards her with two shirts, trousers or any piece of clothing really (just leave out the intimate wear for now though). Don't stammer or appear nervous. Simply ask her which of the two pieces does she thinks is better.

Well, depending on how smooth your conversation skills are (can be developed like everything else), converse with her for a minute. If all goes well, and you've charmed her enough, go for the kill and ask for her number. Rocket science? No!

8. Be the Leader, Decision Maker or Influencer of Your Pack

This again dates back to our evolutionary genes. Women are innately attracted to powerful men or leaders who are in control of their pack. Going back to primitive times, men who were powerful group leaders were seen as highly desirable sexual mates in the mating game. This hasn't changed much since are genetics remain the same.

Women are deeply attracted to men in position and authority at a very subconscious level. So how do you be the man who is in charge of people around him? You can very well demonstrate this from across the table or room.

A simple tip for revealing your leadership prowess is to touch people you are conversing with. Pat men on the back encouragingly. Place your hand on people's shoulders within a brief moment. Do a high five or punch someone playfully.

Well, research in a publication called *Why Women Have Sex* suggests that women often see men who touch people surrounding them as possessing brilliant leadership skills.

They view these men as someone is a position of authority, influence, inspiration, and power. According to women, these are the guys who earn respect.

So something as effortless as making slight physical contact with people around you shows you in a flattering, commanding light.

Psychologically, women have an intrinsic sense of identifying leaders within a group. Men who look authoritative and confident are naturally attractive when it comes to seducing a woman.

To work this perfect leader strategy, you have to smile, stand, sit and walk like you don't care about what everyone thinks.

Work on your alpha male strategy before pulling this off at the next party or gathering. Make yourself look valuable by enhancing your physical looks, leadership skills, and charisma. This will make women yearn for your attention instead of the other way.

Avoid putting anyone, especially the woman you fancy on a subconscious pedestal. You can permanently bid adieu to all your chances of dating and seducing the woman once you place her on a high pedestal. If you are overtly revealing how much you're drooling over her, you are just giving her a secret, unspoken power to dump you whenever she wants.

It is easy for you to lose the woman's respect, affection and subconscious power once you elevate them to a higher pedestal. Make the woman feel that you are too good for her, and she has to make a real effort to get someone as valuable as you.

9. Stay Positive

Well, it's not just a blood group but a way of life that'll make you compulsively attractive to women. If you are in a positive frame of mind (operating with positive thoughts and a feel-good attitude), it'll not miss showing in your body language effortlessly.

You will invariably come across as more friendly, warm, approachable and relaxed.

Can I give you a brilliant technique for maintaining a positive attitude? Have a happy go-to song that you hum to yourself each time you want to feel positive and peppy. This tune should transform you into a happy, feel-good zone while elevating your energy level and mood. Another effective way? Take some time to focus on the aspects you appreciate in others and yourself.

This gives your steps added bounce, and it doesn't go unnoticed by women.

It leaves women wondering what makes you so upbeat, and hey presto before you even say "positive", they've clamored to you to get their share of that radiant, infectious positive energy.

10. Easy yet Subtle Bragging

Well, you don't want to give your dream woman the impression that the entire universe revolves around you by talking only about your accomplishments. However, you have to speak about the goods things too. Otherwise, how are you going to create a favorable and irresistible impression?

The best strategy to get a woman to fall head over heels in love with you is to very briefly and subtly mention your achievements or attributes. Don't linger or dwell on them for too long like it's a huge deal for you. Pretend that these are regular everyday things for you. Another important thing to consider is that you don't belittle her accomplishments to make yours look really big.

For instance, if you have to attend an awards ceremony to collect an award for excellent workplace performance, drop a subtle hint about how you will be busy on the day of the ceremony under some pretext. Similarly, if you are buying a new car or house, mention briefly about how you're busy looking at new homes and cars. Just mention your achievements or acquisitions lightly without focusing on them.

Chapter Three:
Ditch the Friend zone and Get Her to Crave for You

Every guy's worst nightmare is probably getting friend zoned by the woman he fancies. He puts a major spoke in your plans and sends your dream of being in a romantic relationship with her down the awkward friendship alley. Once your friend zoned it becomes really tricky to get into a full-throttled romantic relationship. Here are some of the best tips to avoid being friend zoned by that special someone.

1. Don't be a best friend forever. Some discussions such as her ex-boyfriends, her long-distance potential boyfriend, and other personal things should be off limits. If she's too comfortable sharing these details and using your shoulder to cry on, you are her BFF before even realizing it. mIf you behave like a friend sharing every little detail of her life, you are guaranteed to get friend zoned.

Let her know that you aren't going to entertain discussions about other guys or play relationship agony aunt to her. She'll get the hint if she's perceptive enough.

2. Don't agree with her all the time. In their bid to please a woman, guys often turn into doormats. There's no need to take her to a café or restaurant of her choice all the time to engage in an activity she enjoys. You can do what you want to do for a change or take her to your favorite restaurant.

Following her around like a smitten dog will make her treat you like one. Retain your own unique identity and personality, while still being around for her. If you keep yourself at her beck and call all the time, you'll be friend zoned in no time.

3. Be Attractive Mate. One of the biggest reasons people end up being friend zoned is unfortunately that they aren't attractive or desirable enough to the person they deeply dig. The induce feelings of comfort, reliability, and security without inspiring attraction, seduction, lust, and chemistry.

Groom yourself well. Wear clothes that suit you. Improve your body language. Smell great. Learn to engage in a flirty and stimulating conversation. Act a bit coy in the presence of your crush. When you increase your sex appeal, you are less likely to be friend zoned.

4. Give thoughtful gifts that you would give only special people. Ditch the neckpieces, clothes and rings that require little imagination, and opt instead for something that holds more relevance in her life and shows her how special she is to you. She should know you are keenly tuned in to her interests and passions.

In place of jewelry, gift her tickets for a concert she's been mentioning. It could also be an online course she's wanted to pursue since long or a personalized plushy of her favorite cartoon character. If she's a photography enthusiast, you could gift her magazine subscription for a photography related periodical.

Customizing gifts is a wonderful way to let her realize that she's not like everyone else and that she deserves these special and exclusive gifts.

5. Be bold and simply ask. Another huge reason guys get friend zoned is that they are scared, uncertain, hesitant and more passive while approaching a woman. Many times they believe they aren't good enough for someone. Since the view themselves as just good enough to be friends, the woman starts viewing them in a similar manner. People who think someone is too good for them to use the "just good friends" approach because it isn't emotionally risky and calls for less disappointment.

Do not chicken out when it comes to asking her out and end up saying something else to avoid a potentially awkward situation. Be the Prince Charming that you are or you'll end up being Hamlet. Ask confidently and charmingly, without sounding pushy or sleazy. An invitation for coffee or lunch isn't a huge deal anyway. No guts no glory, follow the adage and you should do well lads.

Don't settle for anything else if your intention was to get into a romantic relationship out of a sense of insecurity. Some guys use friendship as a sneaky back door entry to make their way into a woman's heart rather than facing outright rejection. Avoid all this, and make your intentions clear upfront. If she isn't interested, hold your head high and find someone else. If you still feel you have a fair chance by being friends first, make a decision accordingly. However, it always helps to be bold and simply ask a woman out.

6. Make plans without her. This is a sort of twisted way to make her realize that you have a life without her and that your world doesn't revolve around her existence. Make new friends, hang out with a group of like-minded folks and go out more often without her. If she knows you're always wrapped around her little finger whenever she needs you, she's likelier to friend zone you.

Make yourself unavailable periodically, so that she realizes that if she wants to spend more time with you, she needs to commit to a more serious relationship. Feeling a wee bit neglected will make her claim her spot as your girlfriend.

7. This one's slightly sneaky but worth trying. Give her the impression that you have plenty of girls swooning over you or other options to consider. This way she'll think twice about friend zoning a great guy a losing him to someone else. She may even fear to lose you as a friend, and quickly seal the commitment deal.

8. Treat her like a woman, not a buddy. While it can be tempting to be backslapping buddies before taking it ahead, don't ever fall into the trap. If you treat her as one among the guys, you won't be able to escape the friend zone.

Treat her exclusively and she'll return the favor. Differentiate between the way you treat her and other man and woman friends. Let her know she's special or you. While you should be chivalrous towards all women, make it clear that you do not shower attention on every friend in that tiny black dress. Throw in stealthy glances her way. Pay lavish compliments about how wonderful she looks in a dress (appropriately, don't go overboard). Wait for her reaction and witness if she blushes.

Grab her hand gently while opening doors, direct her to the seat while pulling a chair for her, tuck a hair lock behind the ear, nudge her knowingly and yes hug her frequently. It's also good to tickle her periodically to get the chemistry boiling. Remember to stay respectful while doing all this since you may earn the sleazeball moniker faster than you realize.

9. Try talking when she's all by herself. Don't try to hit on her when you both are surrounded by a bunch of friends. Turn on your charm mode and impress her to the fullest when you get an opportunity. Say something subtly suggestive like, "Just when I was excited about spending time alone with you, these guys pop out of nowhere!" You're hinting at wanting to be alone with her and making her laugh all the same. Leave her perplexed if you're joking or dead serious.

She'll get the idea that you like spending more time alone with her. Make an effort to spend more time together, without really formally asking her out.

10. Do an attitude analysis. How do you appear to others? No one wants to deal with sad sacks and whiners. Don't moan about everything from the global economy to the rude cashiers at the local supermarket.

You need to be charming, happy and sexy. If you cry all the time, you'll only get her shoulders. If you laugh, well you may move a little below shoulders (wink wink). People always enjoy spending time with those that make them feel happy, positive and inspired. Switch your attitude from negative to positive if you think you're being friend zoned way too many times for your own comfort.

11. Develop a sort of sexual tension between the two of you. She should go beyond viewing you like the cute little friend who is always around her. There has to be a magnetism or attraction to make her ditch the platonic friendship stance and move you into the romance zone.

Get a bit touchy-feely with her without awakening her inner defense. Make flirtatious comments, touch her a little and make frequent eye contact. For instance, while watching a film together, put your head on her shoulder casually. Try grazing your hand against her while reaching for the coffee. These tiny physical gestures may trigger her senses, and make her perceive you in a new light.

If she catches you staring at her cleavage, laugh hard, apologize and make it a point to tell her you just couldn't resist it. Throw in a few tasteful innuendos here and there, and you're less likely to get friend zoned.

Little things like looking directly into her eyes when you're saying something significant or holding her by her waist can go a long way in setting the momentum for sexual chemistry. Caress her cheek, brush your hand against hers lightly, kiss her on her forehead, and rest your hand on her thigh – small gestures like these can go a long way in establishing a run up to a more intimate connection. She'll soon realize that you're into her in a more romantic way.

12. Find out from mutual friends how she feels about you. They can generally offer wonderful insights about her interests and state of mind. Common friends can also play cupid and help you two dive into a romantic relationship if things go smoothly. They may also be able to advise you about whether it is a good idea to take things ahead or you're putting your friendship in trouble. Have the drop subtle hints about how the two of you look cool together or get them to put in a favorable word for you.

Chapter Four:
Solid Techniques for Controlling a Woman's Mind and Emotions

If you want to seduce a woman and get her to bed, you have to be able to control her mind and emotions, while making her feel comfortable. Making her yearn for spending more time with your needs more than just regular pampering or opening doors for her. It is about connecting with her at a subconscious level by applying a host of psychological strategies.

Psychological strategies, manipulations, and persuasion don't always imply sneaky tricks to lure and emotionally destroy women for your own benefit. If used positively, it can be used for helping you both get into a mutually fulfilling and gratifying relationship. Here are 10 little-known yet brilliantly effective strategies when it comes to controlling a woman's mind and emotions.

1. Touching For Creating Attraction

If you don't want to get friend-zoned dear friend, by all means, work hard towards developing some kind of sexual tension with the woman you've just started dating. Cruel as it sounds, women often make up their mind within a couple of dates (sometimes just one) about guys they want to friend zone and those they are sexually attracted to.

You need to work with touches just right to build the perfect sexual chemistry or risk blowing it up. It shouldn't come across as desperate or negative, all the same, you don't have to be a limp player who is afraid to make move when it comes to revealing his fondness for a woman. Don't start grabbing a woman too early on in the dating period.

Stick to light touching during the first couple of dates. Begin with hugs, brushing lightly against her arms and leaning or sitting close to her. Lightly brush your arms against hers and let go immediately. Tap her hands or palms lightly and again let go. Don't linger the touch for long. It should be brief enough for her to crave more of it.

You'll quickly gather how comfortable a woman is with your touch by reading her non-verbal signals. If she pulls off or backs off instinctively, she may not be very open to the idea of touching at this stage in the relationship. However, if she smiles, appears relaxed and seems to be having a good time, that's a definite signal she digs your actions.

There's no common yardstick for what you can or can't do in the touch department during the initial few dates. You have to be perceptive enough to understand what the woman desires and make your moves accordingly. Slow, smooth movements are appreciated by women. Don't rush things or be rough with a woman. Chances are you'll never see again in your life.

Breaking the physical touch hindrance isn't a big deal if you do it right. Once you've spent many hours together as friends or dating partners, there's a comfort level that makes it easy for the woman to relate to you.

Start gently by offering a goodbye hug that doesn't linger for more than a few seconds (3-5 seconds). Judge her reaction to know how comfortable the woman is. If she squeezes back tightly or holds you for long, she may just be ready to move to the next level. Similarly, reach out to her hand and brush against it gently. If she grabs your hand tightly or quickly intertwines her pretty fingers in yours, the woman is into you.

Each time you're parting ways tell her something like, "Alright sweets, I feel like a good bear hug today. Give me a nice goodbye hug and then gently proceed to hug her for a couple of seconds. Make it warm and affectionate, and not like all you want to do is feel her breasts or brush your hardness against her. Give her a few seconds to enjoy the feeling, but make it brief enough for her to yearn for it in the future.

Flash her your most dazzling smile after the hug and confidently in a way that's unique to you, "hey, do you realize how beautiful/gorgeous you are (avoid saying seductive, sexy, hot, etc. unless you've reached that comfort level with her)" Add I really dig/like you in the end. This tells her you're after more, and interested in taking it to the next level.

It is easy to break a woman's unspoken touch barrier if you know how to be charmingly flirtatious. Hold a lady's hand and lead her to the bar. Place your arm lightly on her lower back. The idea is to get her comfortable to your touch.

2. You Are Being Tested All the Time

There's no escaping the fact that women are almost always testing men. She's almost always looking for different ways to understand what's going in your mind or your intentions. For instance, if a woman is deeply attracted to you, she may pretend that she doesn't really dig you just to see your reaction/response.

What she wants to establish is that you are a confident and self-assured individual who isn't afraid to hold himself even in the face of rejection. This makes you a highly appealing man in her eyes. Don't get bogged down by her lack of attention or indifference to you. Hold your position throughout your interaction without appearing fazed.

It's a very primordial, instinctive and evolutionary thing for women. If your confidence crumbles or shakes, the woman doesn't view you as being worthy of a male or holding a masculine position. It is easier for her to play the role of the protected. Well, what do they say about making her feel like a real lady? It simply allows women to be more feminine around a man who is powerful. When a woman feels innately feminine in your presence, she will inevitably be turned on by your masculinity.

Ensure that you come across as confident and not egomaniacal. There is a thin line yet the huge difference between the two, especially when it comes to presenting yourself to others. Confidence is deeply rooted in being comfortable in your own skin, and with what you are doing. An ego-driven or egomaniacal personality, on the other hand, fundamentally stems from insecurity or negative self-emotions. Bragging is a huge no-no when it comes to seducing or attracting a woman.

Keep things cool and subtle. Humility makes you sexier. Remember, guys who are innately comfortable in their skin are likelier to impress women than show-offs who operate from a point of jealousy or insecurity. Well, six-pack abs will help your cause but they aren't a necessity.

3. Keep 'Em Guessing

Don't reveal or make your intentions clear almost immediately. Even if you really dig a woman and attempted to tell her straight off, hold back for a while. Women love drama and an element of suspense. Mix your actions by doing both – showering her with attention as well as acting aloof at times.

Just ensure you don't end up confusing her. Keep her guessing about your feelings for her. If you make her too comfortable and fuzzy, she may end up losing interest. It's alright to keep them slightly perplexed without confusing them much. If you've just begun dating someone, act totally into her one moment and nonchalant the next. This is enough to send her mind into a psychological tizzy that keeps her guessing. The sneaky little trick can keep a woman on her toes, and drive her insane enough to keep her hooked!

Playing with her emotions shouldn't be misused or viewed in a negative light. If used well, it can be a perfectly workable strategy for winning your dream woman's affection and establishing a powerful emotional connection. For instance, act supportive one moment and slowly detach yourself in the next. This may appear mysterious or confusing in the beginning. However, later, she'll find herself magnetically attracted to your positive side.

4. Capture Her Senses

Well, much as you're in denial about this, physical attractiveness goes a long way for getting a woman to go to bed with you. Make it a sensory bonanza for her by increasing your attractiveness quotient. Wear comfortable and well-fitting attire in a color that flatters you. Sport a haircut that looks chic, well-groomed and suits your face cut. Smell good, as you're going to be remembered by your smell. Don't make it a very overpowering scent. Keep it is nice and subtle, yet compellingly fragrant.

Research has consistently pointed out that the most critical factor when it comes to awakening a person's sexual desires is smell. This is because pheromones are responsible for triggering sexual desires. Once you are able to influence her sensory experiences, it is easy to charm her.

A study conducted by the University of Management in Singapore revealed that women are highly attracted to men with broad faces since it demonstrates a powerful and masculine persona. I know what you're smirking and saying there, how can I change the shape of my face dude? Nope, you can and don't have to alter the shape of your face. However, you can use tricks to make your face look broader. For instance, you may want to grow a beard or develop some facial muscles by working out in the gym. Women love strong and powerful men, and some physical features convey just that.

Physical attractiveness attributes play on a very subconscious level to attract women. They facilitate or support your body language or non-verbal attraction clues to make you appear insanely irresistible to women.

5. Smile, Smile, and Smile

A smile conveys affiliation, relation, and affection. It is a sign of taking to someone instantly or being attracted to a person. Flashing a genuine smile communicates confidence, positivity, and lovingness in the mind of the person you're out with. Don't expect a woman to jump straight into bed with you as soon as you flash your pearls.

However, it will set the tone for a friendly and affectionate relationship that can lead to bigger things. Once you've established a warm relationship rapport, it is easy to move to more intimate and advanced touch strategies. Psychologically, you're showing your interest or affection for the woman.

6. Maintain Eye Contact

Maintaining consistent and unwavering direct eye contact is the key to displaying your interest in a woman. It not just depicts supreme confidence but also reinforces your intention to seduce the other person, thus establishing a ground for taking the woman you desire to bed. Holding continuous eye contact during a conversation is a psychological sign of attraction. It also works on a physiological level.

When we establish eye contact with someone we really fancy, our pupils start dilating. Even if a person doesn't instantly notice your dilating pupils, at a subconscious level they catch the signal. This only attracts the person further to us. Keep in mind that you don't overdo it or the other person will start feeling uncomfortable or freaked out.

Whatever happens, avoid looking down every now and then. Nothing is unsexy than a guy who keeps shifting his glance to the floor. It makes things come across as awkward and uncomfortable.

Research has proven that looking down constantly can have a negative impact on your and the other person's mental state. Keep things positive by fixating your gaze on the woman you desire. She'll be flattered and reward you with equal attention. Making continuous eye contact can be a great seduction tool, more so if you can add a seductive smirk and raise your eyebrows a bit while doing it. Mighty irresistible? You bet.

7. Practice Active Listening

Much as many mistaken dudes like to believe, impressing a woman isn't about talking nineteen to a dozen until she needs a pill to cure her headache. It is as much about listening attentively to a person to win her affection.

Unlike men, who are more to the point, women love to have extended and long-drawn conversations. They are high on details and the backdrop of every subject/topic they are discussing. If you want to charm your lady, listen keenly to everything she's saying. Offer small acknowledgments that you are listening to her intently.

It can be anything from a nod to a simple yes to exclamations – whatever suits the situation and communicates to her that you are listening to her or completely immersed in the conversation.

One of the most important things when it comes to listening to a woman is to hold back your advice and suggestions. Bite your tongue if you have to but don't offer suggestions or solutions. Much as you want to make her life simpler, simply hold back from giving any advice unless asked for.

Men often share their problems to get solutions, whereas women share their problems simply to talk it out with someone who understands. They are not necessarily looking for guidance or expert advice or someone who treats them like they know nothing. Hence resist the urge to play agony uncle and just listen to her.

Empathize with her, show understanding/concern and just let her know you're there if she needs anything. Don't offer her a 10 point strategy to combat the problem, because you'll end up creating a new problem for yourself.

Listen with interest to stories about her buddies or something she found funny. You don't have to be a yes man and agree with everything. Put your point across in a gentle and non-offensive manner. At times, repeat what she's just said to let her know that you are actively listening.

Avoid talking excessively about yourself. It's alright to give a brief introduction to your background, education, career, hobbies, etc. However, don't go overboard with details about yourself. Again, keep your eyes glued to her. Avoid looking at other women or talking too much about them. Ensure you focus on the woman you're with and make her feel special. You need to give her the impression that she's the only one who matters. And for god's sake, put that phone away when she's talking.

Listen to what your partner is saying. Read between the lines to understand the underlying feelings and intentions. Sometimes, your direct approach may catch them off-guard. They may say something you really don't want to hear. Encourage them to express themselves honestly.

There are several reasons why people may be averse to the idea of our commitment, including personal insecurities, bitter relationships or marriages in the past, childhood experiences related to their parents' bitter relationship, perceived loss of freedom, greater responsibilities and much more. Listen to the other person to understand their concerns. Even if you both want to be in a relationship, your reasons can be completely different.

For example, your partner may want marriage for practical and financial reasons since it makes sense to run a single home then two. On the other hand, your partner may want to get married because they want someone to come back and talk to. Your reasons may be practical, while your partners may be more romantic.

When you talk frankly and honestly about the idea of marriage and commitment, you'll discover diverse perspectives and expectations. Of course, if you are bringing up the subject of commitment, you will be speaking more in the beginning. However, once you realize that the other person is replying to your questions, listen. When you direct the conversation, you are preventing your partner from sharing her truest feelings. Instead of speaking honestly, she will most likely tell you what you want to hear.

The same is true for hearing something you may not like. Listen carefully to her reasoning. For example, she may want to be a relationship but desire to be more financially secure before she gets into a serious relationship. She may want to focus on their career before dating seriously or settling down. If you finish the conversation without letting her share her take on it, you may start believing that she doesn't want to be in a relationship with you at all, which is not the truth at all.

Eliminate the scope for misunderstanding by listening keenly to what the woman is saying.

8. Appear Taken

While this is another sneaky, back-door technique, it can work wonders when it comes to drawing the woman to you like a magnet. Women are biologically wired to go after men that their competitors' desire. It sort of validates the dude's greatness when other women like him too. Women are almost always concerned about how others react to their acquisitions, which is why they need a bunch of girls in tow when they go shopping or even picking a gift for someone. Validation about their choice is important for them from an evolutionary and psychological perspective.

Thus, when someone appears like he is already taken, they tend to feel a sense of validation that the guy is indeed worthy enough of their affection. However, there may be a downside to this too. Many righteous women may prefer staying away from you if you appear taken. They don't fancy treading into someone else's territory.

9. Recognize a Common Ground

One of the best strategies for getting a woman to like you or feel a sense of belongingness/affiliation for you is to identify common ground. Talk about something you both have in common to create a comfort level that can take things to another level. It can be anything from shared moments to hobbies to favorite sports teams to political affiliations. Establishing a common ground makes it easier for you to seduce a woman.

If you gather early in the conversation that a particular topic completely lights up her face, keep dropping it within the conversation every now and then.

Appealing to a lady's sense of humor is almost always the best way to get her to sleep with you. It will invariably up your chances of getting the woman you desire to hop into bed with you. Ever wondered why the nearly scary looking Russell Brand has earned so much success in bed? Just Ensure the lady is laughing with you and not at how ridiculous you are.

Clowns aren't a turn on for women, however, men are comfortable and confident enough to display a clever sense of humor are insanely appealing. Even when you are being humorous, don't try too hard to recite lines from the latest best-selling pick-up manual. Make it sound natural and unforced. It should come across as intrinsic to your personality and not something that requires too much effort.

Put the woman at ease by treading in the domain of subjects she appears to be comfortable with. Making a woman feel relaxed, positive and comfortable is the key to get her to open up and talk about more intimate things. Get her to laugh or keep her glued to the conversation by asking a couple of interesting questions that get her talking.

Make it a mix of spontaneity and planned questions to avoid conversation lulls and awkward moments. The best advice when it comes to impressing a woman is to try to be yourself unless you're an absolute idiot. Then try to be less of an idiot.

10. Apply Fractionation

This is another effective psychological technique used by seduction ninjas. It claims to make women fall for you in as little as 15 minutes or less. The technique is deeply embedded in hypnosis, with inspiration from the theories of both Sigmund Freud and Carl Jung.

The psychological technique involves taking women through an intensely emotional roller coaster to build a strong rapport. Fractionation is known for equipping men with plenty of seduction powers, which helps them enjoy a lot of success with the fairer sex.

Though known to be a highly effective seduction technique, fractionation is looked down upon many as being manipulative and unfair to the woman. It is controversial for being an amoral, dark and unethical seduction technique, similar to brains-washing. It's more like a dark hack and should be applied with discretion.

If you really want to understand fractionation, look at any of the soap operas. They take the viewer through an emotional roller coaster ride with a steady stream of suddenly positive and negative emotions. The audience thus becomes heavily invested in these heart-wrenching emotional sagas. Now you know why women love soap operas!

Fractionation is a mind control technique that involves a combination of voice, hypnosis, words and body language in order to elicit a strong emotional reaction from a woman to persuade her to get into bed with you.

It beings by building an emotional bond by getting her to trust you and open up to you. Ask lots of questions that demonstrate you are one of her league. Later, weave a powerful conversation that triggers strong emotional ups and downs. It can be as simple as initially asking her to describe something that makes her genuinely happy, and later, the saddest moment of her life or something that she deeply fears. Repeat the same sequence, and she'll be smitten.

When women experience positive and negative emotions in a short span, they are sold. Add your own unique aura (conversation skills, personality, and body language) and she'll be melting in your arms. This isn't rocket science but a simple psychological premise.

When an individual (especially women since they are intrinsically emotional) is subjected to polarity (the brain is subjected to a series of feelings such as pleasure followed by pain followed by another sequence of pleasure and pain), it leads to a powerful emotional rapport. You're mentally enslaving her. However, caution against using this technique negatively. It may end up creating a lot of trouble in your and the woman's life.

Here are some instances of creating polarity.

"It feels so wonderful to have your best friend by your side through the ups and downs of life, right? I had the best buddy anyone could ask for. One fine day she just became sick and passed away all of a sudden. She was simply gone, without any warning.

Have you fallen in love with a person almost immediately and felt a deep connection? Like you know you just know from within that it's meant to be forever. I lived through that feeling once. We grew close so quickly. Only a few weeks after we got together, Faye died in a car crash. I mean she just left me and went."

See what I've done there? Built a soap opera like the emotional graph to take your woman through a clear high (happiness), followed by an equally compelling low (sorrow). This helps her experience a deep psychological bonding with you.

If used right, this method can bring a woman in your control in no time. Fractionation is potentially more effective than the "secret seduction sauce" used by sneaky pickup artists. Bear in mind one hazard – it is impossible to undo the effects of this technique once it is applied. Once a woman has been psychologically enslaved with this method, leaving her like a hot potato will cause her immense psychological damage.

Therefore, tread with extreme caution and use this strategy ethically, positively and responsibly. You want to impress women not scar them emotionally for life.

11. Enter Her Comfort Zone

When you're alone with the woman, sit physically close to her. Act like you really didn't notice your physical proximity. If you've only been flirting with her, this is the time to get physically and subconsciously close to her. You are symbolically and literally entering her personal space to build a kind of sexual chemistry.

If she's simply seeing you like someone to flirt with, you need to show her you mean business. Don't make her feel uncomfortable by plonking yourself a little short of her lap. That's not the point. The idea is to show her that you are sexually interested in her, and want to take things to the next level.

Once you enter her space, make an attempt to lightly touch her arms or fingers. Keep your hand lovingly over hers. Slowly wrap your hand around her waist to create a feeling of belongingness and intimacy.

Psychologically, you are entering her space and making her feel comfortable with the idea of sharing her space with you.

One surefire way to winning a woman's affection (and eventually landing her in bed), is to build an intense rapport with her. Begin by making her feel easy in your presence by picking subjects that you know she is familiar with. Once you've grabbed her attention, and have her hooked, tease her lightly and appear playful. Ensure you keep it harmless and don't reveal right up to that you are attracted to her. The strategy is to simply draw her closer and later quickly move away to leave her gasping for breath. It's the same scientific, magnetic principle, where there's plenty of attraction when unlike poles meet.

Chapter Five:

Little Known Secrets for Opening the Key to a Woman's Heart

Attracting highly desirable, loyal, respectful and loving women (I meant just one having all four qualities and not four different women, just in case, alright jokes apart) can be as simple and complex as you want to keep it.

You may have married for 40 years and still not know what drives a woman, and you may be a rank newcomer in the dating game and ace it completely.

It's like one those search engine algorithms (only more complicated and unpredictable), you really don't know what will work to rank your web page on Google and what will not work. The search engines have their own set of complex, secret algorithms (based on several factors) to assign a rank to each page.

Women's algorithms can beat Google's hands down. You never know what will and won't click with them.

However, despite the complicated algorithms we still have people keenly studying Search Engine Optimization (SEO) to rank their pages high on search engine results. Similarly, there are some little-known WMO (Women's

Mind Optimization – okay I just made it up) secrets that can help you map out their desires, and take the highway into their heart.

This book allows you to plunge into their brain, to understand how women think, feel, desire and express, which can eventually help you dive head-on into their heart.

Men and women are essentially wired differently due to a large number of factors including genetics and evolutionary science. The way a man perceives a particular situation and reacts to it can be drastically different from a woman's reaction to the same situation.

 It's not about right or wrong (which is the biggest fallacy we commit), it's just that we are manufactured and upgraded (for the tech-savvy millennials) differently. The operating system is a bit different in both, which is why both the genders function differently, and both are exasperated that the other "just doesn't get them."

When you understand these basic differences and secrets about how a woman's thought process is wired, you are more equipped to impress her. You gotta have to master the rules of the game if you want to ace it, right? Nope, I am not referring to attracting women as some sort of a game for the alpha male. All I am suggesting is to come out tops at something you need to know the rules at the back of your hand.

And I aim to do just that here. To share with you all the proven strategies, little-known secrets, practical wisdom nuggets and much more that armor you up (did you just read that amorous?) for not just attracting the woman of your dreams (or fantasies whatever), but also gaining her love, respect, and loyalty.

I want to make you the ultimate relationship ninja or love doctor (not really Alex Hitchens from Hitch who guides several men to woo women they desire with a magic formula only to be tongue-tied when it comes to his striking a conversation with a woman he desires) who is effortlessly charming with women, knows how to talk to them, understands what they truly want and earns their unwavering loyalty.

Yes, there is a magic formula and secret algorithm at work, but if you look carefully enough, the code can be easily cracked. Demystifying the feminine mind is by no means a piece of cake, but it isn't a herculean task as well. Once you understand the dynamics a pushing a woman's hot buttons (no it isn't what you think it is) – you're well on your way to earning the love, respect, admiration, and faithfulness of the woman you desire.

Put that gaming console aside, grab a can of beer and prepare to be pleasantly surprised and shocked as I unveil some of the most interesting and fascinating insights about the fairer sex.

Wooing a woman is akin to tiptoeing through an intimidating minefield. One faulty move and it can end up as a disaster. Once she's attracted to you, put a plan in action to win her affection and respect. There are winning tactics that you should follow before simply throwing caution to the winds and proposing to her. Here are some secrets to conquering a woman's heart (probably the toughest conquest in the world, even Alexander would agree!)

1. Keep Her Guessing

If she figures our each tiny little thing about you and predicts every move, you'll stop being interesting for her. Avoid predictability to retain an element of surprise. Avoid sticking to a routine like wishing her every morning or checking how her day was at the end of the day. Send texts randomly throughout the day when she least expects it. Sometimes, when you don't have anything interesting or valuable to say, just don't send any message.

Keep her on her toes guessing. Let her excitedly anticipate your next move. For instance, if you're just bored chilling out a café, get up and tell her to go home and dressed and plan something without revealing the place. When she gets ready, take her to the opera or movies. Heck, even paintballing together can be fun.

Being an enigma is almost always a great way to score with the opposite sex and win their affection. In a bid to try and figure out the real you, she'll spend more time, effort and energy thinking about you. Once you're all comprehended, she won't take time to put the pieces of the puzzle together. It's a nice strategy to leave a bit baffled at times. So get out there, and take that rabbit out of the hat!

2. Be Dependable

Be the unflinchingly dependable dude if you want your damsel. Most women seek out prospective mates they can depend or rely on. Be a man of your words if you truly want to impress a woman. When you declare you're going to do a particular thing, ensure that you do it. This polishes your reputation and presents you as a man of integrity.

Complete things that you can on. Follow through things that need to be finished. Have a bunch of friends vouch for your reliability and dependability. The fact that you are dependable and reliable needs to shine through your actions.

It doesn't matter if you don't ask her directly if you think it'll get awkward if it screams date. Instead, you can plan an outing for the two of you by saying, "Hey, I've got tickets for the latest movie that everyone's talking about, and my buddy bailed out at the last minute. Would you like to join me?" You just asked her out without making it sound like you asked her out.

3. Avoid Being Friend zoned

Sometimes, in a bid to win a lady's affection gradually, guys make the terrible mistake of becoming best friends and then transforming it into a full-blown romantic affair. Nothing can be more quixotic than going from a platonic to a physical, romantic affair. It looks great in the movies, but real life is different.

It's alright to let a woman know from the beginning that you fancy her as a romantic mate. That doesn't mean you push her into a relationship immediately. You're still giving her all the time and space she needs to make up her mind. However, you are only making your intentions clear to avoid confusion and heartbreak later.

Don't try to win her heart deceptively by making your way into her life as a friend. When she's talking about other guys, cut her short and tell let your intention be known by saying something like, "My apologies, I am not discussing other men here. Let's just keep it related to the two of us." You are clearly establishing your intention of getting into a relationship with her rather than offering a brotherly shoulder for her to cry on.

At the same time, do not tell the woman on a first date or even within the first few meetings that you're already dreaming of having six children with her or that you want to buy a home for the two of you. She'll be spooked. Drop hints that you're interested in her in a romantic way but do not appear overbearing.

4. Avoid Games

Games are a hugely toxic way to begin any relationship. Before you know it, to maintain a single lie that you uttered at the beginning of the relationship, you are telling a series of lies until it gets to a point where the entire relationship feels false. If you get the feeling that you aren't in the relationship with a similar objective, back off. Don't just keep playing along to please her.

Don't pretend to be something you aren't or fabricate stories just to seem appealing to the woman. For instance, if you haven't ever been in a relationship don't concoct stories about having been heartbroken in a long term relationship or use other such deceitful tactics to win a woman's sympathy or affection.

Also, don't use the tried and tested technique of playing hard to get. It may work for men but isn't much effective when it comes to women. They often misinterpret playing hard to get as a man's coldness or indifference, which can have them running in another direction. You need to show them you care, and are there for them when they need you if you truly want to unlock their heart.

5. Listen without Offering Solutions

There is a major difference in the way men and women communicate. While women pour out their heart in a bid to gain support, solace, encouragement, and comfort, men share their woes to get solutions. This vast gap in the way both communicate leads to huge scope for frustrations and misunderstanding.

When a woman is talking to you about her problems, resist the urge to play solution-provider. Men are hard-wired to come up with logical, rational solutions for everything. There is an inherent need to play the knight in shining armor.

They are happy to offer resolutions, which they believe is making life easy for the woman they love. However, women don't view it similarly.

They don't want to be told what to do or how to resolve their issues (which they view as nothing but an indication that they can't handle their own problems). A majority of the times they do know what's to be done to resolve it. All they need is a listening ear that listens with judging, offering opinions and judging.

The next time a woman shares her woes with you, bite your tongue hard and resist from giving your opinion or solution, and simply listen. Nod to show her you are acknowledging what she's telling you. Keep the affirmative phrases going. Repeat a few words from what's she telling you. Agree with her by making statements like, "Oh yes, I know how you feel about it" "yes, it must have been tough for you."

Simple statements like these that comfort and support her are enough to help you win brownie points with her.

Golden rule – don't offer solutions until she's specifically asking for it.

For additional brownie points make her feel useful and valuable by asking her for solutions. Share something that happened at your workplace and ask her how she'd tackle it, and in her opinion how should you handle such a scenario. She'll be flattered that a strong, in control person like you trust her judgment in resolving important matters. Also, whenever possible, make it a point to show her that you've used her advice and benefitted from it.

6. Sweep Her off Her Feet

Yes, go the whole hog and do everything to charm her. Women are mighty auditory creatures and soothing words deeply affect them. Notice the smallest things about her like a new haircut or a different nail color, and compliment her on it periodically. Keep telling her how wonderful, irresistible and charismatic she is. Let her realize that she wields a magnetic effect on you and that you go blank each time you see her. Never fail to empathize on inner beauty.

Don't forget to surprise her with small gifts, send her flowers and chocolates when she's least expecting them, and wrap your hand around hers in public. The secret sauce of being the ultimate charmer is to demonstrate to a woman that you truly treasure her, find her insanely desirable and care about her feelings.

7. Be Her Loudest Cheerleader

Each one of us needs a cheerleader to help us step out of our comfort zone when doing our best. Many times we become complacent and stop challenging ourselves or practicing self-development. Be your woman's cheerleader. Inspire her to challenge herself and push her out of her comfort zone. Help her pursue her wildest, most impossible ambitions and goals.

Discover her passions and support them fully. For example, if she's into helping the underprivileged, help put together a fundraising drive or accompany her on her social missions. When other people discourage her, offer unwavering support, and let her know you trust her abilities completely. Reach out to her and solicit her advice on important matters too. To inspire her, you must be driven about your goals and passions too.

8. Overcome Resistance

Look beyond a woman's defenses, rejections, resistance, and complaints. She may simply be trying to test your integrity. Women often do not communicate in a very straightforward manner. They just want you to understand or "get it" without spelling it out loud and clear.

When you comply with her wish even if she doesn't display too much interest in your or keenness in taking the relationship ahead, it reveals to her that you care about and respect her opinion. This makes her feel special, and she'll be likelier to open up to you and trust you. Women don't take too kindly to men who chase superficial rewards like physical appearance or sex. She has to be convinced that there's something beyond her looks that's caught your fancy.

9. Give Her a Unique 'Yours Only' Nick Name

This should be your own unique, creative name for her. Please dump clichés such as sugarbun, honey, and sweetie and opt for something more unusual, which resonates her persona. If she's more sensitive, petite and delicate, give her the name of her beautiful flower that symbolizes her fragility.

However, she's a more solid, determined and assertive soul; name her after a rock unique gemstone. Addressing a person by a special name casts a magical spell on them and helps foster a stronger, more cherished bond.

Also, pick "your" signature song or a song that has deep relevance in your life which best describes how you both feel about each other or a situation that is similar to yours. Master the lyrics of this song, and never leave an opportunity to sing it or play it in the presence of your loved one.

10. Share Something Slightly Personal about Yourself

The best way to get a lady to open up and share little known details about her life is to start doing it yourself. Win her confidence by confiding in her. Let her know that you trust her enough to share some of your most intimate secrets with her.

She'll feel insanely special that you care to share such an important part of your life with her. It can be anything from special childhood memories to ambitions to deepest fears to your weaknesses. Talk about how to get all teary-eyed while watching touching flick.

You can also pepper the conversation with your most embarrassing moments while throwing in some humor. The ability to talk about your weaknesses and embarrassing moments spell confidence, which is very appealing to a woman.

Again, don't brag about flashy cars or accomplishments of family members. The opportunistic gold-diggers may very well latch on to your words, but an independent, strong lady who earns her own money is less likely to be impressed by your net worth. She is keen to know more about you, not your balance sheet.

11. Charm Her with Thoughtful Gifts and Dates

Yes, the chocolates and flowers route may work sometimes, but try to think beyond it by pumping up your creativity. Surprise her with thoughtful and meaningful little gifts that hold a high sentimental value, and leave a huge impression.

Ditch perishable items or expensive electronic gadgets for more evocative items like a portrait on how she looked the first time you met her. Get all the details including her footwear, outfit and hair right. Write a thoughtful note about your feelings the first time you set your eyes on her, and pin it to the portrait.

If she's an avid traveler, put together a handwritten bucket list for each country along with some cute illustrations that best represent each nation. (a guy I knew actually did this and needless to say won the wanderlust femme's heart for life).

Women like to see a spark of creativity in their men. Ditch the hum-drum date spots and think outside the box to create fun memories and adventures together. You don't have to rob a bank to impress the right woman. Go hiking together to the nearest mountains if she's an outdoorsy person. Have a picnic next to a lush waterfall instead of a boring café. Take her to the museum, zoo or pottery making class.

This definitely shows the woman you've put a lot of thought, effort, and originality into coming up with something to impress her, which can completely sweep her off her feet. You can have the opportunity to view them in varied situations to get to know them better.

12. Adore Her for Her Quirks

Everyone has a few things they don't appreciate in a person they want to spend their life with. However, if there are too many such things in the person you desire, that's a red flag. To be able to love a person and live with them, you've got to accept their quirks too. If you can't get yourself to fall in love with her supposed weaknesses or make her feel special/unique about her quirks, you won't break the ice with her.

Saying something as simple as "I really like your freckles, they accentuate your beauty" can help you score big time. This can really elevate her spirits, while also revealing that you adore her for the right things.

I know someone who completely ruined his chances by telling the girl he desired that "he loved her despite the gap between her teeth." A huge disaster. Don't think you're being too saintly by telling her that you love her irrespective of her flaws, it only highlights the flaws. Don't bring attention to their insecurities, help focus on the features that make her wow.

13. Make Her Laugh

Making a woman laugh is one of the best ways to win her heart. You're not releasing the feel-good endorphins but also showing her that you can be a fun, intelligent and witty companion who can keep her in splits for life. Crack a joke when she's feeling slightly down, narrate a funny incident that you witnessed on the way or talk about something amusing that never fails to get your goat. Show your sparkly, witty, humorous side to keep her enthralled.

However, she also needs to know that just because she laughs at your jokes and opens up her heart to you, you aren't going to take advantage of her. Just notice this – if she's laughing at you even when you aren't being funny, she definitely digs you.

Ditch the regular coffee/dinner first date, and do something exciting on your first date that lifts her heart rate. Visit a haunted house, an exciting theme park (with scary adrenaline soaring roller coasters) or watch a horror movie. Exciting dates can forge a stronger connection between you both because it feels like you've experienced something seemingly scary yet amazing together.

Chapter Six:
Dating Tips No One Will Share

There are more pages of dating advice for men than probably the number of women on planet earth, and yet men still struggle with winning a woman's heart. Here is a compilation of some of the best dating tips you can lay your hands on so you don't have to go scouring around finding the secretly buried scrolls about what to please a woman. It's all right here. Just read and start using it right away.

1. Choose a Place That Makes You Feel Comfortable

Dating on familiar territory, where the maître d's and managers/owners know you well almost always helps. Actor George Hamilton once described how he visits some of the best eateries in town in the afternoon when it's not likely to be crowded. He graciously introduces himself to the maitre d' and offers them his credit card. Hamilton later asks them to take a print of the same and instructs them that each time he comes there with different people, his card is to be charged for the meal and a 25% tip.

Once he brings people in the restaurant, the staff greets him and directs him to the table. Once dinner is done he tells people that he's taken care of the bill. Alright, I get you aren't a movie star or celebrity but you get the idea, right? Go to a familiar terrain and you are more likely to impress your date. You'll be in a comfortable space, which will reflect in the way you talk, feel and behave.

2. Think about What You Truly Desire

Who exactly are you? What are your passions? If you're a sports buff who grabs the tickets for the season, do you want someone who hates basketball and prefers to have you home watching every night? A majority of the times men are insanely attracted to the physical attributes of a woman while ignoring the bigger picture. They end up with women who don't dig the life they cherish and then end up frustrated.

Just today, I happened to read the story of a man who loved traveling, while his girlfriend simply hated it. He lost his passport and she helped him find it all around the place with no luck. A few days later she admitted having burned his passport while he was away. Needless to say, the relationship collapsed.

Well, that's not to say every woman is going to be a golf kit or game console burning freak. But let's face it, if something is really significant in your life, ask yourself if you are able to live with a person who isn't as much pumped up about your passion or vision.

Yes, a compromise will be required in any relationship but be clear about it upfront. If you aren't going to give up playing or watching sports, lay your cards on the table in the beginning, and come up with a solution that works for both. If your a lady isn't okay with it, you'll have to take a tough call.

3. Have a Plan Ready

Don't just have a casual go with the flow attitude. Make a plan to surprise the lady on a date. It makes her feel that she's really worth all that effort and planning. Women adore surprises. However, they also want to dress appropriately for the activity/date. So while you can tell her you have a plan, don't spill all the beans on the plan just yet.

Give her clues so she can prepare for it accordingly. For instance, if you've planned a hiking trip or long walks, you can ask her to dress casually and wear comfortable shoes. Tell her you'll be doing something fun post-dinner so wear comfortable clothes and shoes.

If it's a swanky dining venue tell her not to afraid to dress up full throttle. It's like giving her cue cards without giving away the entire picture. Leave things to her imagination. Things will be more exciting if she's kept guessing until the end.

4. Be Your Best Version

Rather than pretending to be something you aren't just to attract her attention, try and be the best version of yourself. There are high chances someone will dig you for who you are and things will be easier for you because you won't have to spend the rest of your life trying to upkeep a lie.

Be a superlative version of yourself. Dress amazingly, smell great, and pay attention to personal hygiene. Smile a lot, crack intelligent jokes, laugh without inhibitions, and most important – listen with rapt attention when a woman is speaking (acknowledge and nod). Display knowledge about a wide range of topics without sounding all-knowing or boastful though. Ask lots of questions to display your interest in the lady.

Confidence is hot, while arrogance is completely not. Understand the difference between being self-assured and haughty. Women don't take too kindly to a man who tries to throw his weight around and attract attention. Drama is best left for theatres. Be your confident, positive, real self, and you'll do well!

5. Do Little Romantic Chemistry Checks

Want to know if a woman truly digs you? Do small and random chemistry checks. For instance, lean a bit ahead subtly and watch her reaction. Does she move away from you or take a sudden step back? If she doesn't resist you leaning against her or leans on you in turn, she may well be interested in taking things ahead.

Don't overdo it though or you'll be sabotaging something beautiful even before it begins.

6. Maintain a Lighthearted Conversation

As a rule of thumb, keep away from controversial topics such as politics or world issues where two people can have opposing views. This isn't the best way to flaunt your intelligence. Women want guys who can have them in splits, and also make meaningful, sensitive conversation. They aren't here to hear you rant about your incompetent boss or inefficient subordinates.

 In the early relationship phases, it's all about having fun. So keep it lighthearted, conversational and fun. Don't dive on into serious issues, where your table resembles a global issues summit.

Also as a golden rule, steer clear from discussing your ex. She's just not interested in knowing about how you feel about your ex or the finer details of your break-up. It will only end up boring her and making things uncomfortable between the two of you. If she approaches the topic, keeps your replies short and to the point, without appearing evasive or suspicious.

Assure her that there's nothing to hide and that your ex is a part of your past for a reason. Give her confidence that what's gone is gone and that you're totally over your ex and want to focus on getting to know her really well.

Another tacky topic is money. It either makes you sound gloating or a non-achiever.

Stop boasting about how much money you have or lament about how you never seem to have enough. It totally ruins things for both as she won't know how to react. Avoid making things awkward and just get to know each other for now. Keep your bragging and worrying for another day, and just enjoy getting to each other.

7. Get an Unbiased Assessment a Female Friend

Dating isn't something that's learned. You're just supposed to know all the rules and ace it without any guidelines.

One of the simplest and most ingenious ways to excel at the dating game is to obtain feedback from an unbiased and well-meaning female friend. Spill the beans about your latest date by talking about everything from your clothes to your choice of venue to the conversations to how it all ended.

The next time you go on a date, trust me you'll be much better than your last romantic outing.

8. Avoid Arm Twisting Strategies

If your date gets even a slight inkling that you're always trying to arm-twist people into having your way, they'll be shooting in the opposite direction faster than you can utter "date." You may want to recommend a particular dish for your date or take them to a restaurant of your choice. However, you sense a feeling of resistance or displeasure, back off immediately. Make gentle suggestions without coming across as dominating or overbearing.

Offering suggestions will make you come across as a well-informed and amazing guy. However pushing those recommendations down her throat will make you come across as someone who always wants to have his way, which is a huge red flag for women.

9. The Good-Bye Kiss

Let's admit it - this is something you've been waiting for throughout the evening. Golden rule – don't force it when the other person isn't too eager. Sometimes women aren't ready to kiss yet, while at other times they are simply too shy or awkward to initiate it even though they may want it.

What's the right goodbye kiss etiquette after the first couple of dates? Well, don't make it like a huge deal. Stay more casual about it and it won't alarm her. If you don't know what to do, simply give her a soft peck on the cheek, while lingering about for a few seconds, after which step back gradually. Notice her eyes. If her eyes still shut, and in close proximity to your face, she most likely wants a kiss on her lips.

However, if she steps back or starts talking immediately, it's a sure sign she doesn't want to take it ahead and isn't ready for the kiss yet. Don't be disillusioned though, she may simply be trying to test you. Be your regular confident and self-assured self, bag a second or third date with her, and she'll oblige sooner than you realize. Some girls need time, and a majority of them try to gauge is a guy truly respects their decision or simply forces his will on them.

10. Avoid Talking Nineteen to a Dozen

Dates (especially first dates) are not really the occasion to wax eloquence about your life and accomplishments. Try and keep it brief and pithy to keep her interested. Don't go on a long-winded rant or hail your achievements in one go. Verbal diarrhea seldom cuts it with women. There will be plenty of opportunities to have future conversations with the right person.

Don't stuff all the food in their mouth in a single go. They'll soon develop indigestion. Pause at the right place to draw a response from her. Pepper the conversation by asking questions. Listen with absolute attention (switch off that phone if need be) when she is speaking. It shows her you are attentive and interested.

11. Follow up Etiquette

Don't say you'll call her if you don't have any intention. It doesn't speak of you in a very flattering light, and it may end up hurting her. Just say, "I had a lovely evening." If you really want to see her again, you really don't need to tell her you'll call her, she'll know once you call. Don't play mind games if you aren't interested in someone.

Also, don't leave too many days between the date and callback if you really want to see her again. It may have worked a few years ago. However, it isn't very effective today.

It's pretty much like the twist on that famous adage, "early to bed, early to rise and your girl goes out with other guys." If you don't contact her within a couple of days, she'll assume you aren't interested in her, and quickly move on to the next person.

Call the woman if you're interested in catching up with her again within a couple of days. Don't sound desperate and pushy. Let it come across as you'd really like to do more fun things together to get to know her.

This will show her you're interested without appearing pushy. Don't expect her to reply to what's up when every other guy is asking her the same thing.

Why would she do it? Don't play slots here. Instead, comment on something exciting that you read on her profile or indulge in some friendly banter to break the ice.

Build the atmosphere for sex rather getting straight to the act. Start by gently massaging her legs, hands, and backs with relaxing oil. Help her de-stress to eliminate tension and pressure from her muscles.

Light up an aroma candle on a table next to the bed. A little warm-up goes a long way to in building the run-up to great sex.

Chapter Seven:
Proven Pointers for Earning a Woman's Absolute Loyalty

The dating dynamics of today's millennials are terribly confounding and complex. Loyalty and faithfulness towards a partner almost seem like a prehistoric virtue that has no space in fast-paced urban romantic relationships. An even bigger challenge than wooing a woman is winning her unwavering loyalty. Getting into a relationship with the woman you desire is easier than holding her attention, keeping her hooked to you, and earning her loyalty.

Accept the fact that woman today are more financially independent, self- confident and aware of their expectations. They seek comfort from being vulnerable by dating multiple men casually and have their options open.

How then do you get a woman who has your back? How do you get a woman to support you unconditionally? How do you get a woman who spots your true potential and is ready to help you accomplish your dreams? How do you get someone who will enhance your life with her love and support? How do get a woman to be loyal and committed to you?

Women seek commitment, loyalty, and genuine marriage material, and they are less likely to give up their quest for finding The One. Be genuine without making exaggerated promises, display integrity at all times, respect them and display your sense of commitment and loyalty to win brownie points.

Here are some proven tips for earning the unwavering loyalty of a woman, and keeping her committed.

1. Don't Order Her Around

The easiest way to put off a woman and send her running in another direction is by using rough language. Make her feel like you're some drill sergeant and she'll desert you in no time. Even if things get challenging or rough, never treat her with disrespect.

Even when you disagree with her, do it gracefully without resorting to name calling or using aggression tinted language. Women are extremely intuitive and sensitive towards verbal signs that demean their worth or make her feel unloved.

If you keep using insensitive language, she'll soon head in the direction of a woman who shows her greater love, respect, and appreciation.

2. Don't Be a Spoilt Child

One of the fastest ways to lose a woman's interest is to be just another responsibility. While you may fancy yourself as a child-man who needs to be mothering and pampering, you may just end up being another responsibility in her overflowing list of tasks. Be reliable, not dependent.

Look after yourself financially, pitch in with household chores and be there or her when she requires help. Don't be her child when she needs a solid and reliable man who can lessen her burden. Be responsible for your work, possessions, health, and hygiene. Don't have her running around the house offering you instructions about how to put your things in order. While it may all seem romantic in the beginning, she'll get tired of doing things for you all the time. Keep your promises.

3. Be a Partner in the Real Sense

This is why most of us are in a relationship anyway- to have someone be there for us and share our life. Help solve her problems, reach out to her family in times of need and take control of situations that are causing her agony. Equip her with tools to deal with her problems on her own.

Whether it is helping with household chores if she's working two jobs or taking care of her sibling while she is tackling a stressful situation with her parents or taking her mostly homebound grandfather out for lunch, help ease out things for her. These are signs of being a committed, dependable and reliable individual, and she'll be likelier to reciprocate with equal love and loyalty.

4. Give Her Enough Time

Neglect the girl of you desire once you get her and you'll send her straight down someone else's alley. It's not necessary to meet her each time she wants to, but make your presence felt in her life. Be around when she wants to talk to you or feels like spending time with you. When you spend more time with her, you come across as a committed person, a keeper who is tuned in to her needs.

She's less likely to ditch the feeling of being with another man when she's given the time and attention she craves. Neglecting your girl will send her running in the arms of a man who values her, and gives her more time and attention.

Several men misguidedly think that winning a girl or getting her to commit has won them the battle when it has only just begun. They become complacent and stop investing effort into the relationship. Some smart pants also think putting a ring on her finger will lock her into a committed relationship. Far from true. The hard work isn't done yet, dude.

5. Be Mr. Right

Some women (just like some men) will cheat on their partners despite the guys putting their best foot forward. It isn't about you, it is about them. However, a majority of the times a woman is prone to cheating if you take her for granted, treat her disrespectfully or have lost touch with your masculinity. Avoid being a wimp and be a man of substance.

Be the kind of man that attracts loyalty. Women dig masculine, protective and dependable men who exude a self-assured aura. If a woman believes you are her strong and reliable Mr. Right, she is less likely to ditch you for another person.

6. Tiny Gestures of Appreciation Go a Long Way

Appreciating your girl in tiny yet meaningful ways is a great strategy for keeping her addicted to you. Thank her for all the wonderful things she does to keep you happy, even if they seem rather insignificant to you. Don't forget to appreciate how amazing the dinner she cooked tasted or how awesome she smells.

Never leave an opportunity to tell her what her presence means to you. In a nutshell – make her feel loved and special. When she feels like the most loved and appreciated the woman in the world, you'll be her magnet.

7. Eliminate Terms and Conditions

In the era of marriage contracts and pre-nuptial arrangements, people have forgotten that at the end of the day these are relationships involving emotions. Step back a bit and empower your woman to be more independent in her decisions and life. Let her make her choices, and never forget to tell her that you'll support her decisions no matter what. A man attracts huge reserves of loyalty when the woman realizes that her man loves her without any conditions.

Avoid making her feel like she has to be a pick between making you and making herself happy. Never ask her to make difficult choices between you and her career or between you and her friends. Always encourage her to take positive decisions that make her happy, and as a loving partner, support those decisions.

When a man constantly asks a woman to make challenging choices or tests her love or asks her to prove her love by giving up something that's important to her, he is sending her sprinting in another direction. Leave important decisions to her, and let her know you've got her back.

8. Their Take on Intimacy is not the same as yours

Don't take it personally or feel jilted if she refuses to get intimate with you each time you desire sex. Women have a greater warm-up period than men, which means they need some forewarning and cannot just jump into the bed and get on with the act. They crave greater intimacy in terms of snuggling, cuddling, touching and kissing warmly.

Women seek comfort, gentle touch and thoughtful gestures over rabid sex. Therefore, hold your horses or whatever else that dying to gallop, and give her time to get into the mood. Avoid scaring her. Caress her hair gently, touch her lips, give her a light peck on the neck, murmur sweet nothings into her ear, talk to her about her day, and before you know it you'll both be having the time of your life. Pushing her will only lead to greater resistance and a breakdown in communication.

9. Inspire Loyalty

If you're too smooth with members of the opposite sex, don't expect loyalty from your woman. It's like planting distrust and expecting growth of loyalty. In her mind, you'll be a jerk who isn't to be trusted, which may or may not be true. Inspire her loyalty by being faithful yourself. Don't give her reasons to doubt your intentions.

Try and include her more in your life, spend more time with her, refrain from commenting on other women in her presence and show her that her happiness truly matters to you. Don't attempt to play to the gallery by dressing up and behaving in a manner that attracts attention. Just stick to doing things she likes. Don't seek acceptance and validation from other women; make her preferences your priority. When you have someone you truly want, why would you go out of the way to please others?

If your words and actions sow seeds of suspicion in her mind, she'll treat loyalty as a cheap commodity too. She'll be more likely to justify her acts of unfaithfulness if you give her reasons to doubt your actions. It's a simple equation really – if you want loyalty, give loyalty.

Be mentally strong, respectful and honest, and your woman will rarely feel the need to look elsewhere.

10. Make Her Feel She Is All That She Wished To Be

One little known (shhh don't spill the secret everywhere please) way to inspire a woman's love, respect, and unflinching loyalty is to make her feel like that she's everything she's ever wanted to be. Every woman has a vision about herself during her growing up years. While some yearn to be perfect mothers, others visualize themselves as artists, corporate czarinas, and even problem solvers.

Irrespective of her primary desires, let your woman know that she has indeed met those goals. Shower her with compliments that are in line with her fundamental goals. Help her get the feeling that she's accomplished those goals or is close to achieving them. Encourage her to take up things she's always wanted to pursue.

For instance, if she's always dreamt of being a travel writer and exploring the world, sign her up for an online travel writing program or get someone to design a travel blog for her. Small gestures like these can go a huge way in pleasing your woman.

Chapter Eight:
Killer Techniques to Keep Your Lady Committed Until Eternity

Getting a woman to fall head over heels in love with you is one thing, and keeping her happy and satisfied is totally another ball game. Earning her love, grabbing her attention, and keeping her hooked requires work. Guess what? The rewards are more than worth it if you invest a little effort into making your queen happy! When you know their hot buttons, it is easier to keep them happy, committed and satisfied.

Here are some of the best-known strategies to mankind (yes, we stole the secret scrolls wink wink) that can have your woman not just swooning over you but also completely addicted.

1. Let Her Know She is on Your Mind All the Time

This is something men never seem to get but it is important for a woman to know she's on your mind 24 by 7. They love to know that if when you both aren't physically together, mentally you're always thinking about her. Never leave an opportunity to reveal this to a woman, and you'll have her eating out of your hands.

Women crave security in a relationship. They are subconsciously intuitive towards signs which indicate that their relationship may be in trouble. When you don't respond to her messages or don't call her while you are away, it creates a sort of nagging feeling about you being emotionally distanced or disinterested, which makes her feel insecure. She may feel like she's not needed in your life.

You don't have to call or message her every 4 minutes, but a simple, thoughtful message like "how was your day?", "hope you haven't forgotten your supplements" and "I am missing your delicious home-cooked meals" can go a long way in keeping the emotional intimacy going.

2. Pour Your Heart Out

Just like men are known to be visual creatures, women are verbal beings. They love it when you open up and confide your innermost feelings. It shows her how much you trust and adore her. It shows her you are confident of her companionship and committed enough to share something that you wouldn't usually share with anyone else.

Make it a point to start the conversation by saying something like you never thought you'd share this with anyone ever but how you couldn't stop yourself from sharing it with her. She'll be delighted (and will do a nice little happy jig in her mind) that there is strong emotional intimacy between you two.

Women dig emotional intimacy more than anything else in a relationship. They want to feel they are emotionally needed, and that they can make things easier for you by just being around. Never miss an opportunity to make her feel you rely on her emotionally. Just don't come across as whiny, clingy and dependent.

Learn to maintain a fine balance between being emotionally balanced and leaning on her shoulder or support. She doesn't want to deal with a whiny kid, only a man who connects with her emotionally and feels better after speaking to her.

3. Boost Physical Intimacy

Making a woman happy in bed goes beyond giving her multiple orgasms. It is about developing a deeper connection and emotional bond through pleasurable acts. The next time you climax, instead of heading to the bathroom, hold her warmly and let her know how lucky you feel to have her in your life.

One thing women really abhor is men who simply get up and leave after ejaculation. It makes them feel less valued and more used.

Women seek to be emotionally turned on too for enjoying a mind-blowing climax. Let her know how much you love her, and pay her a genuine compliment about for the day like how wonderful she looked while going to work or what an amazing dinner she cooked despite being tired post work.

4. Disagree Respectfully

No amount of flowers and chocolates is going to help if you are plain disrespectful and indulge in name calling during disagreements. The difference of opinion happens in the best relationships so there's no denying the fact that you both won't agree to everything.

Stop treating arguments in relationships as a contest where there has to be a clear winner. When you ditch that mindset, you'll learn to come to a compromise which will make her love and respect you even more. Addressing disagreements constructively is the sign of a mature man.

For instance, if you both are traveling together and she's an absolute outdoorsy person while you are a homebound (or hotel bound) sloth, keep a few days aside where she can explore the outdoors while you watch a movie.

 You can also go do things you both enjoy doing (lazy lunch at an outdoor café) or split between having her way one day and yours another day.

There may be other disagreements like she may want to meet your folks but you may not be ready for it yet. Work a compromise where she can start by meeting your sibling for lunch instead. Make her understand that you don't want to rush into anything, and that's its best you both to savor the journey of the relationship slowly but surely. Put your point across without offending her.

Chapter Nine:

Online Dating Tips That Can Change Your Love Life Forever

Okay, so aren't exactly Don Juan reincarnated, and have to work really hard at attracting women. No sweat!

The dynamics of social and romantic relationships have changed with the internet. There are plenty of chances for meeting and connecting with interesting women with common interests and values.

Online dating offers plenty of advantages. For one, you don't have to deal with the anxiety (or jitters) of approaching the woman face to face. Also, you can screen potential dates before investing any effort into knowing if they're right for you.

If you're a man with a rather busy schedule, online dating can be a real boon.

With some luck and a solid strategy, you should be able to be the ultimate woman magnet. Here are some of the most effective online dating secrets for men.

1. Shine up Your Profile

Like any other dating scenario, first impressions are vital on the internet too. Just because someone can't see you physically doesn't mean they aren't judging you or forming an opinion about you. Never forget that your profile is being held under a woman's microscopic vision, which means making a solid impression within the first few seconds will earn you greater rewards.

Face it or fume, but women have a far greater choice when it comes to online dating than men. This means you're playing in an extremely competitive field. She's probably scanning ten other profiles along with yours. Scary as it appears, you don't have more than 5 seconds to make a favorable impression or be dismissed.

Much as you fancy yourself as an alpha male, refrain from using a username that flaunts your sexual prowess or a deeply nerdy passion that many probably won't even understand. Don't come across as boastful. Women see this as highly clichéd, uninteresting and immature.

Keep a genuine, sincere, earthy and witty name. Use your first name in your user handle to make it more personal and garner greater responses. Women are more likely to respond to an "Aaron007" than something shady like "Pimpbossguycandy" or "alphamalelongnutz."

I know you're laughing but you won't believe the kind of names these hyper-fertile minds come up with.

Don't include hackneyed stuff like "I love to have fun" or "live to the fullest" or "I love outdoors and animals." It will put her snooze mode on. Show some personality dude. Get that opinion, wit, and sarcasm flowing. Be creative and throw in a unique persona.

Don't shy away from standing out even if it borders on quirky or edgy. Make your profile a fun spoof of some of the most ridiculous clichés circulating in other dating profiles. Women will dig your imagination and out of the box thinking.

Avoid flaunting your wealth, status or income. It may appear counterintuitive, especially if you're successful and financially well-settled. However, it pays to be humble and confident, not cocky and arrogant. You can post pictures of enjoying your wealth without directly referring to it. Include photographs of yourself in exotic locations if you are a frequent traveler.

If you're passionate about a hobby and spend lavishly on it, don't be afraid to include pictures of it. Add a sense of mystery to your profile by withholding something. Let her thought bubble has "what does this man really do?" inscribed all over it.

The bio section of your dating profile wasn't meant for you to give vent to your hidden author and write a biography. The ideal length is between 60 – 300 words long. Anything above that and you'll leave her yawning. Keep her excited for a face to face meeting. If you reveal every little detail about your life, you aren't leaving anything to her imagination.

Give her the chance to figure you out by being an exciting and challenging jigsaw puzzle.

The woman's imagination will make you more interesting than a long-winded essay about how amazing you are. When you say how wonderful you are, it loses its appeal. Show her how wonderful you are rather than boasting about it yourself.

Dress in something that matches your personality not something that reinforces cheesy, unimaginative stereotypes like a power suit or rock legends tees. Women appreciate a little bit of subtlety in everything since they like some things to be to their imagination.

Be more descriptive and specific. Learn the fine art of creating an impact using a minimum number of words. The primary objective of online dating is to find someone with shared passions and interests.

It will help if you are more specific or descriptive about your interests. Instead of stating that you love music, mention the specific genre of music you dig. Rather than saying, sunsets fascinate you; describe where and when you witnessed the most spectacular sunset.

All this adds more dimension to your profile, which makes it stand out. It also gives your date more fodder to reply with something meaningful and interesting.

Take the time and effort to draft a profile that genuinely reflects your persona. There's no need to be pretentious, yet it's important to inject some humor and fun into the profile.

You can get important and high-value points across in a playful manner too so that she can better relate to it. It just shows her how you don't take yourself very seriously and has the ability to laugh at yourself too. Self-deprecating humor is a sign of confidence, self-assuredness, and high self-esteem.

When you poke fun at yourself, you come across as less vain and more confident. It's no secret that women dig funny, interesting and witty guys who can keep them enthralled. Don't be funny throughout the profile (if that isn't your dominant personality), but pepper a few one-liners or sarcastic, self-deprecating remarks here and there to make the introduction more interesting.

2. Add the Right Profile Picture

Nope, the smiling profile picture works wonderfully well for when it comes to attracting men but women are hard to please creatures. Studies have pointed to that fact that women aren't really attracted to men who are flashing their pearls in photographs.

The ones that gain most traction are pictures that have the man looking proud or brooding. Research has also indicated that a man's left profile is considered most attractive by women. Take a picture of yourself staring to the right, and give a lower glance or brooding look. Watch the responses pour in as women go weak in their knees.

Women don't like to view men as vain creatures smiling into the camera. Most women dream of a man who is intense and focused. So a headshot of you smiling into the camera may not get as many responses as you playing pool, and intently focusing on making the right shot. Now that's really for a lady. They like their men to be focused and ambitious, so ditch those smiling selfies, and click yourself focusing on something.

Sites like match.com allow you to post 26 photographs. However, you won't be tried if you fail to use every byte provided for your pictures. Stick to 6-8 good and accurate (non-misleading) pictures. You only increase her chances of finding that one unflattering picture and not responding to you by including a ton of pictures. Stick to a few good ones, and give her the opportunity to see you in person.

I see tons of profiles of guys with their male buddies. Why boy why? You already have too much competition to contend with, and you're making it tougher on yourself by standing alongside other men and invariably being compared to them. Imagine women thinking, "He's kind of cute, but his buddy is cuter. Oh! How is wish I could get to know his friend" Learn the fine art of cropping unwanted competition.

Also, while a few lifestyle, travel and hobby related images are cool, this isn't Facebook. Women want to see you, not the scenery where you took a fantastic photograph.

This is one amazing and a little known secret that can work wonders. Always keep your last photograph interesting. It gives the woman something to begin a conversation. This can be your hobby or lifestyle related picture. Pose with your pet dog or post a picture of you volunteering at a camp – the idea is to give the other person an interesting thread or topic to base the conversation on. This is what makes you unique, and gives women a reason to get in touch with you over others.

3. Playing Hard to Get Doesn't Work Well Online

Cruel and unfair as it seems, more men than women exist on online dating portals, which means women can afford to be picky. Don't get disheartened if you don't elicit responses, especially for beginners.

It may take time to understand the dynamics of online dating. The easiest, sneakiest and most effective way to learn the tricks of the trade is to browse through profiles that generate maximum responses and try to include similar tips in your profile.

When you aren't getting the responses you desire, try tweaking your introduction or use another profile picture. Don't wait to be approached.

Be more proactive, and reach out to like-minded women with short, interesting and teaser-like introduction emails.

Playing hard to get may have worked once upon a time. However, in the fast-paced online dating world out of sight is out of mind. Don't expect a woman to chase you if you are more evasive or take time to reply. She'll quickly move on to the next profile, while you'll be left brooding. If you like someone who has approached you, reply promptly.

4. Keep it Baggage Free

Unless you've been living in a cave, chances are we've all had our share of drama, baggage, relationship issues and a history of exes. Don't mention in your introduction that you were on the verge of a breakdown after your previous relationship went haywire or that your ex was the biggest scum you ever encountered. These aren't the details you should be sharing with potential dates. Not yet. Everyone one has a past and is aware that you may have had a past too. There's just no need to be explicit about everything upfront.

5. Get Things Rolling

I get it; you aren't comfortable sending a full-on flirty message to someone who has caught your fancy just yet. You're still clueless and tongue-tied about how to approach her.

It's absolutely alright to simply like a photograph or a profile just to express your interest without being too direct about it. She'll know who you are when you approach her in the future.

This is termed as exposure effect in psychology, which simply means that people automatically develop a preference for elements that induce a feeling of familiarity in them. If a woman notices you liking her photo, she may become more receptive to receiving your message. However, you should continue following up to set things in motion.

6. Set Yourself Apart

How many times have you heard "I love music, meeting people and traveling" and silently cringed? More than half the world loves music and travel. How does that make you unique or unusual? However, living in 20 states across the United States, taking voice modulation classes and having taken a sabbatical from work for wildlife photography is something that makes you stand apart from the crowd.

These are interesting nuggets that we wish to know about you. Please ditch the "I work hard and play harder" clichés, and come up with something more original that conveys who you really are.

7. Write Original Openers

Do you realize how annoying it is to get slammed by hundreds of messages waxing eloquence about how angelic they look or how their eyes speak volumes? Another non-creative message about her eyes, nose, lips and angelic face and you'll get the boot. In the world of online, it helps more to know what not to write than what to write.

How do you expect her to reply to a "hey, what's up?" when she receives hundreds of messages from clueless and unimaginative guys every day. Are you giving her a reason to reply to your message? Write a message about something interesting that she's mentioned on her profile.

Indulge in some lighthearted, teasing or friendly banter to break the ice. Show her some unique persona if you want to stand out from the others. Don't dive right into offering sexual favors. Unless she's a really desperate or opportunist being, she's going to gather all her friends and enjoy a good laugh at your expense. Be original, fun and gentlemanly in your approach.

8. Partner, Not Shopping List?

Seriously, I mean are you kidding me? Are some folks looking for partners or grocery items? The gigantic lists they come up with can put a supermarket's inventory to shame. I am looking for someone who is between 5'7 to 5'11 feet tall, lives in the heart of Houston, and has very short hair and blue eyes. What are you doing? Casting for a film? They are a huge put-off. It makes you sound like a finicky, control freak. It appears like you're looking for a replica of your ex-lover or someone you've always fancied.

While it's alright to have your preferences in place, don't go specific when it comes to superficialities like the person's race, ethnicity, location, physical features, etc. They make you sound like a very hollow and picky person. Be more open and flexible to meet different types of people rather than shutting yourself off to a few folks.

We all have some non-negotiables like you may not want to date someone who has been married earlier or someone who deeply into religious practices. It is alright to mention these things but making your profile look like a made to order partner shows you in a not so flattering light.

Chapter Ten:
Pointers for Getting Your Crush Completely Hooked

Well, so now that you've slowly established your intention to take her to bed or even slept with her, how do you get her hooked to you or earn her unwavering loyalty so she doesn't look elsewhere. I've got your back here too. Here are some of the best tips to get your woman addicted to you.

1. Pamper Her

This one's no secret sauce yet it's baffling how many guys never get it. Women love to be pampered and showered with undivided attention. Cook a simple yet delicious meal for her (bonus points if it's her favorite food). Play soft music in the background. Decorate the room with colorful flowers.

Keep a bottle of her favorite wine ready. Make it a memorable evening by enjoying a stimulating conversation. Be a smooth talker, and infuse your conversation with plenty of humor and compliments. The wine will get you both to feel giddy-headed and get things heated up in bed. Pamper her with unexpected gestures and she'll be floored enough to be completely hooked to you.

2. Be Sauvé

It doesn't hurt to be fashionable or dress nattily to remain desirable in the eyes of your woman. Make a constant effort to be more polished, suave and romantic. Always yourself more valuable, and act like you know your true worth. We know by now that women crave the attention of alpha males with high self-value who are desired by many

It's the world's worst kept secret that women are fundamentally driven by their emotions and not by logic. Don't make the mistake of trying to use rationale with a woman to influence or persuade her. Instead, appeal to her emotions by focusing on romance, affection, and demonstrations of love.

3. Tell Her You Are Thinking About Her

Most men never understand the importance of letting a woman they have to know that they are thinking about her. Show a woman how she's on your mind 24 by 7, and you'll have her positively enslaved. To retain her affection, you have to show that you think about her even when she's not physically there with you. This one tip will have her swooning over you and more often than not attract her loyalty.

Women are innately emotional creatures who crave attention and security. They are subconsciously highly territorial in nature when it comes to relationships, and can intuitively identify certain signs that indicate the relationship is under threat. Don't ignore her calls and messages, which send a feeling of being emotionally distanced. This doesn't mean you drop her a message every 5 seconds. Sending simple yet thoughtful messages (inquiring about her day or telling her how you kiss her home-cooked meals or reminding her to take her medicines) throughout the day can make the relations work in the long run.

4. Introduce Her to Your Friends

A great way to get a woman hooked to you is by introducing her and including her in your gang of buddies. This is your way of showing her you value her enough to be included in your inner coterie.

Be warm and affectionate with her in the company of your friends. Allow her to feel a sense of belongingness with the group.

Compliment her about something that's unique to her. She'll be floored on being showered with affection and respect publically and will reciprocate by keeping you happy and staying loyal to you.

5. Use the Power of Words

Women are high on words, verbal creatures. Why do you think they listen so intently to soulful lyrics of musicians such as Tracy Chapman and Phil Collins? Their words are rich with emotions that tug at your heartstrings. Words are a deep way of connecting with people because they awaken certain sensations inside you.

Write old-fashioned and intimate love letters to your woman. Move your woman with the right words. If you master the art of using the perfect words at the perfect time, you'll get to bed and keep them there faster than you can imagine. Just ensure to keep it genuine so it doesn't sound contrived or falsely flattering.

Chapter Eleven:

Fantastic Tips for Getting a Woman to be Sexually Excited and Yearn to go to Bed with You

Congratulations! You've progressed to the next level and successfully established a comfort level with the woman of your dreams. There is an unmistakably warm camaraderie and a slowly building sexual chemistry. It's time to go for the kill and have roaring sex with the woman you fancy. Here are ten incredibly effective tips to get a woman sexually excited and insanely desperate to make love with you.

1. Set the Stage

I'll let you in on another powerful secret to get a woman to sleep with you. The chances of a woman getting physically intimate with you are directly proportional to how much she relates to you or spends time thinking about you. Occupy a major chunk of her mind share and you've occupied her bed space too.

The guy a woman thinks about for a majority of the time is the guy she is most likely to go to bed with. Don't you want to be that dude? One pro tip is to send her psychologically and subconsciously addictive texts. There are tons of ways to get her interested in you by sending texts to trigger psychological addiction. Ask her about her day or if she needs a little pampering. How about a relaxing body massage? A couple of spa treatment probably?

Compliment her about how attractive she was looking in a particular dress she wore on the date last night. Make her feel like she's the one.

2. Foreplay Fun

Scary as it sounds, this will make or break your chances of going to bed with a woman. Don't undermine the importance of foreplay in getting a woman sexually excited. While it is relatively easy for men to be sexually drawn to an attractive woman, women are wired much differently. They don't simply fancy jumping in bed with an attractive guy, but need someone they can relate to on a more emotional level.

Women love a demonstrative man who isn't afraid to reveal his fondness for them in the form of lingering touches, long smooches, and intimate hugs. Establish a close connection through these affectionate gestures before enjoying torrid sexual intercourse with her. Just because you are ready to rip apart her clothes and make love, don't assume she is.

Use these effective erotic gestures to win her before going for the kill. Cupping a woman's face is a sign of deep admiration and adoration. Start by rubbing /kissing her lower neck. Whisper sweet nothings into her ear. Kiss her lightly on her shoulder. Stare into her eyes as much as possible. Try to move slowly, smoothly and gently from neutral zones to her erogenous zones, instead of simply penetrating her.

Concentrate on the woman's erogenous zones to stimulate her yearning for sex. Make an effort to touch, kiss, fondle/caress and lick her in specific sensitive, intimate areas of the body. Not everyone responds to sensations/touches in the erogenous zones similarly.

Certain zones tend to be more sensitive for some women than others. The two primary erogenous regions for a woman are her feet and head. Give her a gentle foot massage or kiss her lightly on her head. Kissing during foreplay can involve licking, seductive sucking and biting. A woman's lower back, abdomen, and inner thigh region are also extremely sensitive to intimate touches. A majority of women derive great sexual pleasure from being touched in these erogenous zones.

3. Move outside the Friend Zone

If you're like most guys, your number fear when it comes to a woman you fancy is to pray hard she doesn't friend-zone you or see you simply as a good friend.

The tricky part is a majority of the time if you're friend-zoned, it is challenging for her to view you in a romantic, non-platonic manner. Here are my expert tips to avoid the dreaded friend zone.

Again, play up the competition and validation element. Give the idea you have several women desiring you, and a woman will seldom want to give or friend-zone someone who plenty of others desire.

If you don't want to be her best friend, don't act like one. Don't play agony uncle or have innately personal conversations about her ex-partners. If she becomes too comfortable with the idea of having such personal conversations with you, she'll be running for your shoulder to cry on each time tragedy strikes, and you'll befriend zoned faster than you realize. Avoid sharing every intimate detail with her if you don't wish to be friend-zoned.

4. Work on Your Kissing Skills

Kissing is a huge turn on for both men and women. There are volumes of books dedicated to the fine art of kissing because that is indeed the stairway to get a woman excited about going to bed with you. If you get this right, the woman will be yearning to go to bed with you. Too often, men are close to sleeping with a woman they desire and ruin it with their awkward kissing skills, which is a big turn off.

Start by holding a woman close to you. Linger on with the gaze for a few seconds longer than usual. Look straight into her eyes, and speak to them. Brush your lips lightly against hers for a few seconds and pull back. Do this a few times teasingly, before holding her lips with yours. Slowly, bring in your tongue, and place the tip of the tongue on her lips. Don't start drooling or indulge in sucking her lips. This is all the more important if it's your first kiss as a couple.

Keep your breath awesome. Bad breath is a huge turn-off. If you have even a slight inkling of stinky breath, chew some mint or gum to keep the foul breath at bay before going on a date. A golden kissing rule – always keep your eyes open while kissing. It strengthens the connection subconsciously and gets your girl even more excited.

Always leave the lady wanting more when it comes to kissing. You'll get clues to her kissing style in the way she responds to your kissing overtures. How does the woman kiss you back? If you're perceptive enough, you'll get a good idea about what she truly enjoys. Just keeping doing more of what she's leading you to do.

5. Be the King of Romance

The journey from friendship or dating to landing up in your bed can be quicker if you present a more romantic side. Of course, the idea is not to pretend to be someone you're not. It's no secret that women adore men who swoon over them and sweep them off their feet with romantic gestures. Read the woman carefully to understand what she craves for, what impresses her and when you should stop.

Some women love when you flirt with them, while others are easily offended and take even harmless flirting as a sign of you wanting to go to bed with them. Don't give the impression that you are attempting to manipulate or control their feelings for sex, while also being in control of your own feelings.

Showing respect, old-fashioned chivalry and courtesy help men win a lot of brownie points with women. Notice how women have butterflies fluttering in their stomachs in the company of men who display a more gentlemanly and civilized behavior. Few things are hotter than good manners.

Women dig men who appreciate them and demonstrate the right emotion towards them. All some women want is attention, and are quick to jump in bed with men who shower them with plenty of attention.

6. Create Sexual Tension

At times, a woman will be extremely horny and ready for roaring sex without you having to try too hard. Yet, you need to work towards building sexual tension in the beginning.

What exactly is this sexual tension that is referred to throughout the book? Sexual tension is nothing but an exciting feeling occurring between two people who feel a compelling physical attraction for each other but physical intimacy is delayed owing to their unique circumstances, environment, personality, etc.

For instance, even though a woman is strongly attracted to you sexually, she may not want to come across as too easy to get laid. Similarly, two people may be working together in an organization that doesn't really encourage personal relationships between co-workers. Sometimes, either of the partners may already be committed to someone else, and may not go beyond foreplay or making out.

Building sexual tension by delaying gratification is a great way to keep the woman begging for sex. Women really dig the exciting feeling of releasing the sexual tension built up over a period of time. They love the idea of building up tension through kissing, making out and touching each other. Don't undermine the importance of creating sexual tension when it comes to enjoying torrid sexual encounters.

You can enjoy a few brief and exciting make-out sessions before finally taking her to bed after building plenty of sexual tension. You may want to send a host of pre-sex texts that establish that you are attracted enough to want her in bed.

Avoid telling the woman straight off that you want to sleep with her. It may just ruin the excitement you've been trying to create over a period of time. Allow her to feel a strong connection with you before she decides to take it to another level. Play it gently and slowly, warm up before going full throttle in bed and ensure she's in the right mood to get intimate with you.

Having a slightly dirty conversation is also a good way to build sexual chemistry. How do you start? Simple.

Pose a question that appears innocent but paves the way for something crazily dirty. Before you both even realize, you will be pinning for each other. Some men like to set the pace for excitement by indulging in phone sex before going for real sex. It's a great way to understand your girl's sexual fantasies and appetite for sex! Watch out for the verbal clues she offers while talking about sexual acts.

7. Create the Perfect Setting

When men want sex, they become pretty immune to everything around them. Women, on the other hand, are more sensitive to the environment around them. Distractions such as loud sounds, dazzling lights or even dirty bed linen can put them off from the act of sex.

Simple things like turning off the television, changing unclean bed sheets, playing soft music in the background and dimming the lights work wonders in awakening their sexual desire. Make the place aglow with soft candlelight (preferably nice smelling aroma candles), since low light and scent both can act as active triggers for lighting a woman's sexual desires. Use bright furnishings in the bedroom.

Candles not just create an exciting and intimate mood but also go a long way in making the woman feel less insecurity (especially if you haven't gone to bed with her before) about getting undressed or revealing her body.

Colors such as red, orange, purple, etc. convey passion, energy, enthusiasm, and strength. Bright red linen or curtains can wonder in the bedroom.

These are all stimuli that act at a subconscious level to stimulate a woman's deep-seated desires. It talks to a woman at a very subconscious level that you care to put in a lot of effort to get her excited about the prospect of having sex with you.

Music is an important part of the set-up. It needs to resonate with the night's seductive and sexy theme, however, don't make it too loud or distracting. Concentrate on your togetherness than playing a personal favorite playlist. Dude, you may dig death metal but doesn't appeal to a majority of women. Some types of music can accentuate the romance or intimacy, but most are a huge distraction or turn-off for women. Ask her what type of music she prefers to score big with her.

8. Demonstrate Patience

Nowadays every girl is wary of being used for sex and then dumped like a hot potato for the next hottest thing. It is easy for them to assume based on past experiences that all you want to do is go to bed with them. These negative thoughts playing in their mind may make your charm appear more manipulative and fake, even if you genuinely care about her.

Try not to come across as aggressive, pushy or affected when things go according to how you desire. Be prepared for unexpected things. Stay calm, gentle and sweet even in the face of rejection. Once the woman sees you as someone who has the ability to be nice despite not having his way, she's likelier to get rid of the defense walls built around her. It may simply be her way of testing your patience or how serious you are about making an effort to win her affection. Women can play a lot of hard to get games to try your patience. If your tide through these tactics confidently and patiently, you'll win her respect.

Historically, psychologically and evolutionarily, physical intimacy is a big deal for women. They treat it with probably the same measure of seriousness that you would treat say purchasing a new car or signing up for a new home. They don' just sign on the physical intimacy papers without you giving them a compelling reason to do so. And you know only too well once a car buyer walks away from making a purchase, he almost never returns. It is the same with women.

Display patience when it comes to understanding the woman's ideas and values related to physical intimacy.

9. Read Her Fantasies

Don't make sex a cut and dry chore or mechanical task for your dream woman once she looks ready to go to bed with you. Before you take her to bed, try to understand her fantasies. Avoid freaking out if it includes Brad Pitt.

 Instead, make it work to your advantage. Role-playing and fulfilling fantasies are one of the best ways to get women hooked and keep the sexual spice intact. Things won't go stale if you are creating various exciting and stimulating sexual situations in the sack.

One amazing tip for triggering a woman's sexual fantasies is to initiate things or get things to spice up in the most unexpected places. Of course, no one's asking you to get into trouble with the authorities but a little frisky behavior goes a long way in getting someone to feel a compelling urge to go to bed with you.

150

It is easy for dating couples to do the expected or slip into a routine/standard cycle (meeting, dating, hooking up, getting hitched, etc). Try to approach her for making our or hooking up in a totally unexpected place.

Identifying and meeting a woman's need is the best bed to keep her hooked to you in bed. When you go to purchase a car, does the smooth-talking salesman simply flash a sports car and inquire if you liked it enough to buy it? No right?

He'll first inquire if you want a car that gives great mileage or one that accelerates fast or one that gives you good control while driving through rougher roads. Later, he'll match it with your requirement, and you'll be like "wonderful, this is precisely what I wanted." Learn to personify what others seek in you. If the woman you're with seeks a lot of adventure, excitement, and independence, do your darnedest best to give her exactly that.

10. Don't Focus Only on Sex

Don't make sex your only intention with the woman you desire. If you seem too pushy or easy, it won't be a challenging prospect for them to go to bed with you. The secret sauce is to be the exact opposite of what most are (yearning for sex). A majority of men are simply operating with the intention of getting a woman to go to bed with them. When your approach is different, you stand out.

You move away from the desperate trap to act more in control of getting the woman to do what you want. Don't try to persuade her to sleep with you. Rather make her feel like she should convince you to go to bed with her. Chances are women make up their minds pretty quickly about guys they want to get intimate with. Even before you can think "sexy boobs" to yourself, she knows whether she wants to share them with you.

Women are used to guys drooling over them. If you make it a challenging prospect for them to go to bed with you by acting like you're not very keen on sleeping with them, it'll make the prospect even more exciting for them. Do something that women are not accustomed to, and you'll have them eating out of your hands. Don't make yourself an easy conquest.

Demonstrate through your actions that you're not going to be an effortless acquisition and that she has to work really hard to get you. This makes the proposition of wooing you even more exciting for the woman.

Conclusion

Thank you for purchasing this book. I genuinely hope you enjoyed reading it. I also hope the book has offered you a bunch of actionable, practical and interesting tips to not just attract women but also keep them addicted to you forever.

The next step is to simply use all the wisdom described in the book and transform your love life. Apply these little-known yet astonishingly proven strategies to be the ultimate lady magnet. Now that you know how women think, act and feel, use these psychological tricks to earn their love, respect, and unwavering loyalty.

Lastly, if you enjoyed reading the book, please take the time to share your thoughts by posting a review on Amazon. It'd be greatly appreciated.

Here's to being a self-assured, confident, charming, fun and irresistible woman magnet!

www.ingramcontent.com/pod-product-compliance
Lightning Source LLC
Chambersburg PA
CBHW070706250726
48662CB00001B/288